Health and Safety in Schools

Health and Safety in Schools

Barry Stock
FIOSH, RSP

Formerly Principal Safety Adviser,
Inner London Education Authority

Croner Publications Limited
Croner House
London Road
Kingston upon Thames
Surrey KT2 6SR
Telephone: 081–547 3333

Copyright © 1991 B Stock
First published 1991
Reprinted 1991 (twice), 1993
Second edition 1993
Reprinted 1994

Published by
Croner Publications Ltd,
Croner House,
London Road,
Kingston upon Thames,
Surrey KT2 6SR
Telephone: 081-547 3333

British Library Cataloguing in Publication Data
Stock, Barry
Health and safety in schools.
1. Great Britain. Schools. Health & safety
I. Title
371.70941

ISBN 1-85524-228-1

Phototypeset by Intype, London
Printed by Whitstable Litho Printers, Whitstable, Kent

Contents

Introduction

Health and safety is an area where governors, headteachers, safety representatives, staff and parents share common objectives. Minor differences of opinion may exist as to how these objectives can best be achieved but generally there is every reason for everyone concerned to be pulling in the same direction.

The law imposes the responsibility for making satisfactory arrangements for health and safety on management while making provision for safety representatives to monitor their effectiveness on behalf of the staff. Safety representatives are also expected to encourage cooperation between the headteacher and staff where the promotion and development of health and safety measures are concerned. Given an appropriate level of commitment by everyone involved, this framework allows all objectives to be achieved.

The greatest problem, perhaps, is in keeping things in proportion. There is a very narrow path to be trod between being complacent on one hand and on the other being alarmist. Straying in one direction will result in unnecessary disruption and wasted resources, straying in the other direction may result in disaster in one form or another.

This book seeks to deal with those issues which experience has shown are most likely to cause difficulties. It largely avoids those specialist curricular areas which have already had the benefit of coverage elsewhere, except where particular weaknesses have been exposed or new requirements have arisen.

The first chapter describes the health and safety legal framework and subsequent chapters explain how it is enforced and applied in schools. The extent of the individual responsibility of headteachers, their deputies and other members of staff is described in Chapter 3. The principles and methods of carrying out inspections and accident investigations are of general application, whether they are carried out by headteachers, deputy heads or heads of department on behalf of the employer or by safety representatives in the interests of their constituents. While these areas are dealt with in a non-specific manner, information is given about the interface between these roles.

It is important that management, safety representatives and staff understand each other's duties, functions and responsibilities as well as their own because it is only by the cooperation and teamwork of everyone involved that health and safety objectives in schools can be achieved.

Second Edition

It is remarkable that less than three years after completion of the first edition it has proved necessary to add some 15,000 words to the original text largely to cover the requirements of new legislation.

The simultaneous introduction of six sets of regulations (the relevant Health and Safety Commission publications contain a total of 275 pages), may cause some concern and confusion. It is hoped that this edition will assist in determining what needs to be done in schools to meet these new requirements.

Where necessary the text has been revised and updated. Lists of further reading have been amended to include recent relevant publications. Additional subjects, such as food safety law, the EC, industrial tribunals and consultants have been covered, and information about legislation "in the pipeline" has been included. To assist in a better understanding of the meaning of "reasonable practicability" the example of a practical system is described in a new appendix.

The Department of Education and Science (DES) has recently changed its name to the Department for Education. To be precise the new title should be used when referring to very recent and future activities of this department, while references to the DES should be prefixed "former" except where publications are concerned. The likelihood of confusion is further enhanced by most, if not all, LEAs having an "Education Department". In the interests of simplicity and clarity "DES" has been used in this edition to describe the government department responsible for education.

The need to tread carefully the narrow path between recklessness and excessive caution described in the Introduction to the first edition is perhaps even more important now than it was three years ago.

Wickham Bishops   BARRY STOCK
Essex

January 1993

Chapter 1
The Law and Related Issues

This chapter briefly describes various legal requirements in respect of health and safety in schools and associated matters such as insurance and compensation.

The interpretation of the law is ultimately a matter for the courts and to form an opinion as to what they might decide requires a detailed and informed study of the exact circumstances involved and of similar cases. Health and Safety Executive inspectors are usually willing to give advice on matters relating to health and safety legislation and its implementation. Advice and opinions on civil law issues are best obtained from a solicitor. Most trade unions are able to provide expert legal advice for their members where the matter in question is work related.

It is sometimes said that prior to the Health and Safety at Work, etc Act 1974 (HASAWA) employees in schools did not enjoy the same legal protection as people working in industry. This is, however, only marginally true. The duties imposed by HASAWA are not significantly different from the duties which already existed under common law. The main change that occurred in 1975 was that certain breaches of the existing common law duties of care, which previously could have resulted in actions for damages in a civil court, became also breaches of criminal law which could result in an appearance in a Crown or magistrates' court.

Civil Liability—Common Law

The "common law" is made up of the body of decided case law of general application that has been built up over many years. It is not fixed, except by the doctrine of precedent which requires a lower court to follow a previous judgement of a higher court. The highest court, the House of Lords, can reappraise its previous judgements and any new decision becomes binding on lower courts. In so much as judges are continually being asked to adjudicate on matters not previously brought before a court, new law is being made all the time. While there are established principles in common law these are applied in the light of current attitudes and knowledge. (What would have been considered reasonable in 1930 might well not be so considered now.)

The decisions that make up common law include those made in respect of the effect of statute law (made by Parliament) on a particular set of facts. If both statute and common law apply in a case but appear to contradict each other, statute law is followed.

Employers' common law duties

There is a long-established duty of care owed by employers to employees not to subject them to unnecessary risk. This duty is a personal one and cannot be delegated. Employers are required to provide a safe place of work and safe plant and equipment. They are also expected to select suitably qualified people to carry out work for them, to provide training where necessary and to provide competent supervision. Employers must devise and implement safe working practices and maintain them by whatever means are appropriate, such as training, adequate supervision, incentives and disciplinary procedures. All these duties are qualified by the term "reasonable care". Employers must ensure that employees know the dangers arising from work and know what the precautions are. They must ensure that the precautions are available and that employees know that the precautions are available. (What is reasonable is what the average person, the famous man on the Clapham omnibus, would consider to be reasonable.)

Employees' common law duties

Employees (and, indeed, members of the public) have a duty to take reasonable care to avoid acts or omissions that it can be reasonably foreseen might be likely to injure someone. They are also required, by implied terms of their contract of employment, to obey the lawful and reasonable instructions of their employer, and to do their work carefully. A breach of the first requirement resulting in injury would constitute grounds for a civil action for damages, while breach of the latter would be a breach of contract.

Injuries caused by carelessness of an employee may well not be the fault of the employer. The law has, however, recognised that an injured employee suing another employee would almost certainly mean financial ruin for one without compensating the other. To overcome this difficulty the principle of vicarious liability is applied.

Vicarious liability

Employers are liable in law for the consequences of wrongful acts of employees if they are committed in the course of their employment. There is considerable case law defining what is meant by "in the course of employment". If, for example, a teacher injured another by pulling away a chair as a joke, vicarious liability would not apply and the perpetrator would be personally liable. Employees must be doing what they are paid to do, even if in a careless, dishonest or disobedient way, for the employer to become liable.

If the employee has committed a legal wrong and the victim elects to sue the employer, the employee does not necessarily evade all penalty. The employer's insurance company may, through the employer, seek an indemnity from the wrongdoer, but in practice such action is normally only taken in cases of collusion or wilful misconduct. In cases where employees are particularly blameworthy the court may order that they pay a proportion of the damages.

In loco parentis and "the system"

Over the years numerous cases involving injuries to pupils at school have resulted in the establishment of common law principles relating specifically to school life.

In common law teachers stand "in loco parentis" so far as pupils in their charge are concerned. This is an easily understood concept which has the great virtue of enabling that which is acceptable in law to be readily determined in all the varied situations that occur in schools. Quite simply, if the degree of care exercised by a teacher is at least as great as that which would be taken by the average, careful parent in the same circumstances, then this legal duty is discharged. A prudent parent, of course, would pay due regard to the age, intelligence and physical competence of the child in question.

3

Headteachers are expected to maintain an adequate system of supervision to protect pupils at all times when the child is in the care of the school. The question of what constitutes "adequate supervision" regularly arises, with demands for an approved ratio of pupils to members of staff to be laid down by the LEA. Whether a level of supervision is adequate in given circumstances will depend on a number of factors, such as:

(a) the age, maturity, usual standard of behaviour and number of the pupils in question
(b) the nature of the activity and where it is carried out
(c) the supervisory ability of the staff.

One experienced teacher might adequately supervise 200 well behaved pupils in a school hall, while a ratio of one teacher to five difficult pupils may be scarcely adequate in more hazardous surroundings.

Headteachers are responsible in common law for the system of supervision because they alone have the detailed local knowledge and professional experience necessary to make proper judgements.

Civil Liability—Statutes

In addition to common law, Parliament intervenes from time to time in order to define in detail minimum standards, or to establish new principles. Examples are the Occupier's Liability Acts 1957 and 1984, and the Employer's Liability (Defective Equipment) Act 1969. The application of these statutes to a given set of circumstances is interpreted by judges using the principles developed in common law.

Employer's Liability (Defective Equipment) Act 1969

Prior to the introduction of this legislation workers injured as a result of defective tools and equipment had difficulty in bringing a successful claim for damages. Employers simply had to show that they were unaware of the defect, that they could not reasonably have known of the defect, and that they had exercised reasonable care in obtaining the item concerned, for the claim to fail.

This Act means that the employer is liable if the defect in question is wholly or partially the responsibility of a third party, whether identified or not. Thus the employee readily obtains compensation and it is left to the employer (in practice the employer's insurance company) to bring an action against the supplier, etc to recover monies paid out, costs, etc.

Occupier's Liability Acts 1957 and 1984

These are important pieces of legislation for schools, defining as they do the civil law duties of care owed by occupiers towards people who come onto their premises. The occupier is the person who is in immediate occupation or control of the premises. All necessary measures must be taken to ensure that lawful visitors (eg pupils, staff, HSE inspectors, parents) are reasonably safe when using the premises for the agreed purpose of the visit. Occupiers are required to take into account that children require a greater degree of care than do adults.

Where contractors are concerned it is not necessary to warn them about dangers which they should, by virtue of their calling, know about (ie occupational hazards) but they must be told about any hazards that are peculiar to the site about which the occupier is, or should, be aware. If, however, the occupier actually supervises the work of a contractor, it is necessary to ensure that adequate safety arrangements are made, although this would probably not extend to telling a skilled person how to do his or her work.

Under s.2(4) of the 1957 Act it was possible for an occupier to avoid liability by putting up a suitably worded notice. The Unfair Contract Terms Act 1977, however, now invalidates attempts to contract out, by notice or otherwise, of liability for death or injury arising from negligence, or for loss or damage to personal property unless it can be shown that it is reasonable so to do.

Prior to the 1984 Act the extent of care owed to trespassers on premises was decided by common law. The position now is that an occupier must take reasonable steps to protect trespassers from dangers on the premises if it is reasonable to do so. This duty may be fulfilled by discouraging people from running the risk by erecting warning notices, by physically deterring access by fences, anti-climb paint, etc. (Occupiers may erect, say, a razor or barbed wire fence but its nature and the dangers of climbing it should be apparent to a potential trespasser; traps must not be set.)

Trespassers whose presence is condoned (eg a blind eye turned towards children using a playground over a weekend) will probably be considered to be lawful visitors and will be owed a greater duty of care.

Education (School Premises) Regulations 1981

These regulations, made under the Education Act 1944, place a statutory duty on LEAs and governors of voluntary aided and controlled schools. S.24 requires that "every part of a school building shall be of such design and construction that the safe escape of the occupants in case of fire and their health and safety in other respects is reasonably assured".

Health and Safety Legislation

From the beginning of the last century health and safety legislation was introduced on a piecemeal basis. Acts, regulations and orders were introduced relating to specific areas of work and even to individual processes. There were inconsistencies in requirements for similar situations in different industries and in enforcement. By 1970, although there were well over 500 pieces of such legislation, none of it applied to about 10 million workers.

There was also considerable doubt about how effective such legislation was in securing health and safety, because each year 1000 people were being killed at work and half a million people injured. Certainly some companies appeared to find it more economic to pay occasional small fines rather than to maintain the requisite standards.

(Although this legislation did not expressly give the right to injured employees to sue for damages for breach of statutory duty the courts held that such rights were implicit.)

The Robens Report

In 1970 a committee was set up by Parliament under the chairmanship of Lord Robens to look at the whole problem of health and safety at work in depth. In 1972 the committee reported back in a document which has become known as the Robens Report.

The report is still of interest because many of the problems considered have yet to be completely solved. It pointed out that 23 million working days per year were being lost through industrial injuries and diseases, at an estimated cost of £200 million, about one per cent of the gross national product. The accident rate had remained more or less constant for several years. It was believed that the root cause of the problem was apathy and that safe working conditions could not be brought about by external

6

agencies such as the law. There was a need to awaken an interest in safety and to encourage employers and employees jointly to tackle the problem in the workplace.

The existing health and safety legislation was heavily criticised. It was said to be "badly structured" and attempts to cover every eventuality had resulted in "a degree of elaboration, detail and complexity that deters even the most determined reader". The law was said to concentrate on the physical aspects of safety such as guards, while in practice most accidents arose from "habits of work, site tidiness, and human error". The report further criticised the arrangements for enforcement, with five government departments running seven separate inspectorates. A number of recommendations were made, including:

(a) replace the mass of existing legislation with a single Act applying to all places of work
(b) replace the mass of detail with a few simple precepts of general application
(c) change the method of enforcement so that prosecution was not the first resort
(d) extend occupational safety to protect visitors and the general public
(e) actively involve the workers in accident prevention procedures
(f) place more emphasis on safe systems of working rather than technical standards
(g) the approach of inspectors should be changed so that "it should be as natural for them to discuss safety and health problems with workpeople as it is to discuss them with management".

Lord Robens' previous experience of safety representatives in the coal industry, where they have made significant contributions to safety over the last century, encouraged him to recommend that the same concept should be applied to all places of work.

The report was accepted by Parliament and the resulting legislation, the Health and Safety at Work, etc Act 1974, received all-party support.

The Health and Safety at Work, etc Act 1974

This Act had three main effects. It imposed general and wide criminal obligations on employers, as individuals and corporately, and on manufacturers and suppliers of articles and substances used at work. Secondly, it gave the new enforcing authority, the Health and Safety Executive (HSE), wide powers and duties, and created a new administrative structure for it. Thirdly, it gave employees the rights to be represented and to be consulted on matters relating to their health and safety.

The Health and Safety at Work, etc Act 1974 (HASAWA) is also an enabling Act, allowing the Secretary of State to make regulations, and the Health and Safety Commission (HSC) to issue approved codes of practice.

S.2 states that it is "the duty of every employer to ensure, so far as is reasonably practicable, the health, safety and welfare at work of all his employees". This obligation is then spelled out in detail in the following subsections. Subsection 2 requires:

(a) the provision and maintenance of plant and systems of work that are safe and without risks to health

(b) ensuring that the use, handling, storage and transport of goods is safe and without risk

(c) the provision of such information, instruction, training and supervision as is necessary to ensure that employees can carry out their work safely

(d) the maintenance of the workplace in a safe and healthy condition and the provision and maintenance of safe means of access and egress

(e) provision and maintenance of a safe and healthy working environment, with adequate facilities and arrangements for employees' welfare at work.

These requirements, all qualified by the phrase "reasonably practicable", are a restatement of the common law duties owed by employers to their employees, but breaches become criminal offences.

(In deciding whether something is "reasonably practicable" it is necessary to assess the likelihood of an injury occurring and how serious it is likely to be, and to balance this against the cost, in money, disruption, etc of precautions that would be needed to avoid it. If a risk is minor and the cost of prevention is great, it would not be reasonably practicable to take those precautions. If, however, the cost is reasonable given the likely consequences of an accident it will be "reasonably practicable" (see appendix). "Welfare" means statutory welfare provisions, such as sanitary accommodation and first aid. "Plant" means machinery, equipment or appliances, including portable electrical tools.)

Subsection 2(3) requires employers with five or more employees to prepare, and revise as often as is necessary, a written statement of their policy with respect to health and safety and details of their arrangements, etc for carrying out that policy. The statement and any revisions must be brought to the attention of all employees.

Recognised trade unions are given the right to appoint employees as safety representatives. They must be consulted by the employer "with a view to the making and maintenance of arrangements which will enable him and his employees to cooperate effectively" in achieving and monitoring the required standards of health and safety (s.2(6)). Subsection 2(7) allows for the establishment of safety committees (see "Safety Representatives and Safety Committees").

S.3 requires employers to conduct their undertakings in such a way as to ensure, so far as is reasonably practicable, that non-employees are not exposed to risks to their health and safety by the work activities. Self-employed persons are required to do their work with due regard for their own and others' safety. ("Non-employees" will range from pupils to contractors working on site.)

The civil duties imposed by the Occupier's Liability Acts have been described. S.4 of HASAWA in effect makes a breach of that legislation a criminal offence. It requires persons in control of premises to ensure, so far as is reasonably practicable, that premises and equipment are safe for people using them for work even though the people concerned are not employees (members of the public, including pupils).

S.5 requires persons in charge of premises to use the best practicable means to prevent the discharge of noxious or offensive fumes or dusts into the atmosphere. ("Offensive" is not defined so presumably this is a matter for subjective judgement. "Best practicable means" is effectively an absolute requirement subject to the limitations of current technical knowledge.)

The legal duties of persons who manufacture, design, import and supply articles (plant, machines and equipment) and substances for use at work are specified in s.6. They are required to ensure, so far as is reasonably practicable, that such goods are safely designed and adequately tested, and that all information necessary to allow for safe usage is provided. Originally, manufacturers, etc were required to consider the safety of goods when they were used as intended and information had to be provided on request. This proved to be unsatisfactory and s.6 was amended by the Consumer Protection Act 1987. The main effect of the amendments is to require manufacturers, etc to take into account risks (such as operator error or inattention) arising from foreseeable misuse and also to take such steps as are necessary to ensure that adequate information is provided to users.

S.7 imposes duties on employees. They are required to take reasonable care to ensure that their acts or omissions at work do not adversely affect the health and safety of themselves or other persons. (This, again, makes a breach of the existing common law duty of care a criminal offence.) They are also required to cooperate so far as is necessary so that employers can comply with any duties or requirements placed on them by any of the relevant statutory provisions (eg the HASAWA, regulations made under that Act and the legislation listed in schedule 1 of HASAWA).

A duty is imposed on everyone at a place of work by s.8. It requires that no person should "intentionally or recklessly interfere with anything provided in the interests of health, safety or welfare in pursuance of any of the relevant statutory provisions". This section applies to anyone over the age of criminal responsibility and this means most secondary pupils. (One prosecution taken under this section involved an employee who used surgical tape from a first aid box to effect a repair to pipework.)

The employer is prohibited by s.9 from charging an employee for anything "done or provided in pursuance of any specific requirement of the relevant statutory provisions" (eg if an employer supplies safety foot-wear because the risk of foot injury is sufficiently great for it to be reasonably practicable to do so, an s.2 HASAWA requirement, no charge may be made. If, however, the risk is not that significant an employer may make a charge, possibly at a bulk purchase discount price. The Education Act 1988 prevents schools making a charge to pupils for the provision of goggles and similar protective equipment).

Ss.10 to 14 authorise the establishment of the Health and Safety Commission (HSC) and the Health and Safety Executive (HSE).

S.15 enables the Secretary of State to make regulations to give effect to ss.2–9 of HASAWA (eg Health and Safety (First Aid) Regulations 1981, Health and Safety (Information for Employees) Regulations 1989).

Under s.16 the HSC can issue codes of practice, subject to the approval of the Secretary of State. (Approved codes of practice spell out how various aspects of the duties imposed by HASAWA may be fulfilled. Failure to comply with an approved code of practice can be used as evidence that an offence has been committed unless it can be shown that what has been done instead is at least as effective—s.17.)

The following sections, ss.18–26, concern the powers of inspectors and enforcement and this subject is covered in detail elsewhere in this book. (See "HSE and enforcement in schools".)

Criminal proceedings are dealt with in ss.33–43. An inspector wishing to institute proceedings must do so within six months of learning of the alleged contravention (s.34(3)).

Where "the employer" is a corporate body (eg a local authority, governors of a voluntary aided school) and an offence is committed with the consent or connivance of members, officers, etc of that body, they may be individually prosecuted (s.37).

S.40 places the burden of showing that all reasonably practicable steps were taken on the person who has been charged. The prosecution is only required to state a suspicion that this might not be so.

The question of an injured person's rights to claim damages for breach of statutory duty where HASAWA requirements have not been met are dealt with in s.47. Offences under ss.2–8 cannot be used to found an action but as previously explained such breaches would also be breaches of common law which would entitle injured parties to damages. The pre-existing implicit right to sue under legislation such as the Factories Act 1961 and the Offices, Shops and Railway Premises Act 1963, which were made relevant statutory provisions under HASAWA, is preserved. It is also intended that breaches of regulations made under HASAWA can be used to found civil actions. However, Regulation 15, Management of Health and Safety at Work Regulations 1992, specifically excludes the use of that particular piece of legislation in this way.

The standard of proof required in criminal cases is "beyond reasonable doubt".

Borrowed standards

In workplaces such as factories and offices, the pre-HASAWA legislation, for all its faults, spelled out in some detail what was expected of employers. The "new entrant" areas such as education were not so fortunate. Managers and the enforcing authority were faced with the difficulty of determining precisely what the generalities of HASAWA requirements meant in practice and in detail in schools. An answer to this problem was seen in the use of the concept of borrowed standards. A school is not a factory, but a school workshop is similar in many respects so the standards and health and safety spelled out in the Factories Act 1961 could be applied. In classrooms people sit at desks doing written work, an activity akin to office work, so the standards of the Offices, Shops and Railway Premises Act 1963 could be borrowed. (This legislation applies directly to the school office.)

This concept must, however, be applied with care. There is a fundamental difference between a school workshop and a factory workshop. In the factory situation the people at risk are adults, many with years of experience gained working in such an environment. Pupils are more vulnerable by virtue of their inexperience and often by their lack of self-discipline. While it is therefore valid to apply the standards spelled out in the Factories Act and associated legislation for machine guarding, lighting, eye protection, etc, this can only be a starting point. It will also be necessary to take additional precautions such as preventing access to moving parts via maintenance panels, having a lockable master switch system to disconnect power immediately from all machines in an emergency and to prevent meddling, and, of course, providing a far greater degree of supervision than would be expected in industry.

Even where school staff are concerned this concept has weaknesses. The Sanitary Accommodation Regulations 1964, which lay down levels of provision for office workers, etc, are applied in the absence of any other standard to staff in schools. However, office workers, unlike primary school teachers, do not have to restrict their visits to a 15 minute break period and the borrowed standard proves to be quite inappropriate.

Although the Workplace (Health, Safety and Welfare) Regulations 1992, (fully in force 1 January 1996), and the Provision and Use of Work Equipment Regulations 1992, (fully in force by 1 January 1997), will eventually see an end to most needs to borrow standards, certain Factories Act associated legislation covering the training of woodworking machine operators and abrasive wheel installers will remain in force and will continue to be borrowed for schools. During the transitional periods of this new legislation it will be sensible to borrow standards from it rather than from that originally intended for offices and factories.

European Community

The United Kingdom became a Member State of the EC in 1973.

Although the Community makes "regulations" and "decisions" it is a third type of Community law, the "directive", which has particular relevance in the field of health and safety. The 1987 Single European Act added Article 118A to the Treaty of Rome. This Article deals specifically with health and safety at work and provides for the adoption of directives by majority rather than unanimous agreement of Member States.

Directives spell out results to be achieved and specify a date for formal implementation. When agreed by the Council of Ministers they become a binding requirement. In the United Kingdom legislation is drawn up to meet the requirements of each directive. The proposed legislation is considered by Parliament (usually by a select committee in each House) before it becomes law.

A typical example of this process is the Framework Directive which deals with "the introduction of measures to encourage improvements in the safety and health of workers at work". It was adopted by the Council of Ministers in June 1989 and was to be implemented by 31 December 1992. Much of this directive was met by existing United Kingdom health and safety law so legislation covering only the outstanding issues was drawn up. The Management of Health and Safety at Work Regulations 1992 came into force on 1 January 1993.

By October 1992 12 directives concerning health and safety had been formally adopted, with many more in the pipeline. It seems likely that in future most if not all new United Kingdom health and safety legislation will originate in Brussels.

A second area of EC activity which will affect health and safety in schools is the harmonisation of laws on product safety intended to facilitate the free movement of goods in the Single Market. Directives made under Article 100A to date include the Machinery Directive and the Personal Protective Equipment Directive. Others are being negotiated. These directives set out essential safety requirements which must be complied with before products may be sold in the Community. Suppliers will be responsible for ensuring that products meet the appropriate standard. It is anticipated that eventually products will be manufactured to harmonised standards published by the European standardisation bodies CEN and CENELEC under a mandate from the EC Commission. When published they will be adopted in the United Kingdom, using a common number (eg EN 7890 will become BS EN 7890 here).

When these directives are fully in force conforming products bearing the "CE" mark will have exclusive access to the United Kingdom market.

Industrial tribunals

These tribunals consist of a legally qualified chairman and a representative from each side of industry. They have statutory jurisdiction over employment matters such as unfair and constructive dismissals, sex and race discrimination and equal pay. They also hear appeals against improvement and prohibition notices issued under the Health and Safety at Work Act, and applications by safety representatives concerning payment for time off for training.

Industrial tribunals are less formal than the courts. Evidence is given on oath but the rules of evidence are not strictly applied. Legal aid is not available, and individuals may present their own case or be represented by a friend or a trade union official. Costs are not awarded except against a party considered to have acted "frivolously, vexatiously or unreasonably". Cases are decided only "on the balance of probabilities" and decisions made do not establish precedents or necessarily follow those made in apparently similar previous cases.

Applications must be made within time limits. For example, appeals against enforcement notices must be made within 21 days, while for cases concerning unfair dismissal or time off for union duties applications must be made within three months.

It is possible to appeal against a tribunal decision but only on a point of law.

Insurance and Compensation

Compensation for injuries

A breach of a common law duty of care or of a statutory duty which results in injury or loss may allow the injured person to found a civil action with a view to obtaining a compensatory award of damages. If it can be shown that the claimant was wholly or partly blameworthy by virtue of not having exercised reasonable care (contributory negligence), the judge may reduce the award accordingly and proportionately.

The burden of proof in such cases rests on the plaintiff. The standard of proof (on the balance of probabilities) is a lesser one than the "beyond reasonable doubt" required in criminal cases.

Damages are a sum of money calculated with a view to putting the injured person back to the position enjoyed before the accident. Of course, no money can really compensate for the loss of good health or a limb, but it is fair and reasonable within the limitations of the system. Such awards are made up of general damages, which cover pain and suffering and future loss of earnings, and special damages which represent provable losses, such as damage to clothing, loss of earnings, etc, up to the date of the trial. Although there is not strictly a "going rate" for a given injury judges do explain how they have calculated the sums involved and similar awards are made in similar cases.

In order to establish a case for action it is necessary to show that a defendant owed the plaintiff a duty of care, that the duty has been breached, and that damage has resulted due to that breach.

In practice up to 90 per cent of such claims for compensation do not reach court. Each day in the High Court can involve the loser in costs of £4000 and it makes sense for the defendant's insurers to avoid the possibility of having to pay both damages and costs by settling out of court unless they are reasonably sure of their case. The costs involved can be a deterrent to an individual seeking compensation unless he or she qualifies for legal aid or is a member of a trade union prepared to support the claim.

Personal injury does occur in circumstances where no one is legally at fault. In such cases compensation can only be obtained if specific insurance cover exists. If, for example, a pupil is crippled in a game of rugby at school where there was adequate supervision, rough play was discouraged and there was no unreasonable disparity in the sizes of the players, there is unlikely to be any legal redress. Parents and staff should be aware that they need to take out personal insurance to cover such eventualities. Some schools arrange for a single policy covering all those pupils whose parents pay an annual premium.

Time limits on actions for damages

The Limitation Act 1980 stipulates that an action for damages for personal injuries must be commenced by the issue of a writ within three years. The three year period runs from the date that the injury was sustained or from the date that injured persons become aware that they have a disease for which they might be able to claim damages. If an injured person dies within the three years, the period runs from the date of death or from the date that the dependants discover their right to sue. Where injured persons are under a disability which prevents action within the normal time (eg the persons are minors or are of unsound mind) the period runs from the date that they are able to bring an action (ie the persons reach the age of 18 or soundness of mind is restored).

This means that if, say, a nursery pupil suffered permanent harm as a result of negligence at school and the parents did not bring an action on his or her behalf at the time, he or she could bring such an action upon reaching his or her 18th birthday, or within three years of that date.

The time limit for actions other than for personal injury or death is six years.

The Act grants the courts discretionary powers to accept late actions where it is fair and equitable to do so.

The Employer's Liability (Compulsory Insurance) Act 1969

It is compulsory for employers to have insurance cover of £2 million against claims for damages by employees arising out of any one occurrence. (Certain large organisations such as nationalised industries and local authorities, whose assets, etc are such as to permit their self-insurance, are exempted from this requirement, as are some small family firms. Voluntary organisatons may also not have such cover.)

The policy also covers claims arising from occupational diseases caused during the period of insurance but where the symptoms have not become apparent until many years later.

To avoid situations arising where employees could not obtain damages and costs awarded to them because the employer had invalidated the cover by breaking some condition of the policy, the Employer's Liability (Compulsory Insurance) Regulations 1972 were made. These regulations do not, however, restrict the rights of an insurer to seek subsequently to recover from the employer monies it has paid out in such circumstances.

Insurers are required to issue a certificate of insurance which employers are required to display where it can be seen and read by all employees. Failure to insure or to exhibit the certificate are criminal offences.

It must be emphasised that this insurance only provides cover in cases where the employee can prove negligence or breach of statutory duty against the employer, or against fellow employees for whose actions the employer is vicariously liable.

Public liability insurance

In addition to the compulsory insurance described above most employers will also insure against claims that might be made by non-employees under common law or statutes such as the Occupier's Liability Acts. Public liability policies typically provide cover against legal liability for injury, loss or illness suffered by non-employees, and loss or damage to their property. They exclude liability arising out of the ownership and use of motor vehicles but some policies may be extended to cover the personal property, including motor cars, of employees; however, usually claims are restricted to cases where the employer is legally liable for any loss or damage.

Further reading

Farmer, D *So far as is reasonably practicable*, Croner 1990
Health and Safety at Work, Croner. (A loose leaf reference book with bi-monthly updates.)
Munkman, J *Employer's liability at common law*, Butterworth 1985
Articles and substances used at work IND(G) 1L (rev), HSE 1988
Barrell, G R and Partington, J A *Teachers and the Law*, Methuen 1985

Chapter 2

The HSE and Enforcement in Schools

The HSE and the HSC

The Health and Safety at Work, etc Act 1974 (HASAWA) established two new bodies to direct and enforce legal matters relating to health and safety.

The membership of the Health and Safety Commission (HSC) reflects the interests of industry, the trade unions, local authorities and the public. The HSC has wide-ranging powers and can, for example, institute research, set up inquiries, and prepare and issue Approved Codes of Practice in respect of ss.2–7 HASAWA and associated regulations. It also formulates policies which are implemented by the Health and Safety Executive (HSE), and local authorities who are responsible for enforcement in areas such as shops, offices, catering and consumer services, but not on their own premises.

The HSE directs and coordinates the activities of operational staff in:

(a) Field Operations Division
  (i) factories, agriculture and quarries
  (ii) Employment Medical Advisory Service
  (iii) specialist inspectors and scientific support staff
(b) Special Interest Inspectorates
  (i) explosives
  (ii) mines
  (iii) nuclear installations
  (iv) railways.

The Employment Medical Advisory Service provides the HSE with assistance in matters concerning occupational medicine. It was established by the Employment Medical Advisory Service Act 1972 which replaced 2000 part time factory doctors with a full time service, with approximately 100 employees. The Service provides guidance and assistance on a wider and more discretionary basis than was previously possible.

The factory inspectorate has a long and distinguished history. It has been responsible for the enforcement of safety legislation since 1833. The HASAWA extended the legal protection previously enjoyed by other workers to people employed in education. The inspectors, in being given a wider remit, were also provided with very considerable powers by the new Act.

HSE inspectors are responsible for the enforcement of the following:

(a) Health and Safety at Work, etc Act 1974 (Part 1)
(b) regulations made under that Act
(c) legislation defined as relevant statutory provisions in that Act (eg Offices, Shops and Railway Premises Act 1963, Factories Act 1961).

Education Service Advisory Committee

The HSE has set up national interest groups (NIGs) for main industry areas such as printing, construction and education. Staffed by inspectors the NIGs are responsible for monitoring the safety performance of their respective areas, for drawing up Guidance Notes, etc on the implementaton of legislation, for the development of policy, for providing specialist advice to inspectors and assisting in the drawing up of draft regulations which are submitted through the HSC to the Secretary of State. Some NIGs also service an industry safety advisory committee set up by the HSC to consider health and safety issues in their respective sectors of employment. The Education Service Advisory Committee (ESAC) is made up of representatives from teaching and non-teaching staff unions and employers' organisations such as the Association of County Councils. ESAC considers the implications for education of proposed legislation, examines problem areas and makes recommendations through the education NIG, and periodically issues advisory documents covering matters that it has identified as being of concern.

Powers of Inspectors

Inspectors carry written warrants which detail their powers. They must produce these on request and if they are unable to comply they may be refused entry. (Impersonation of an inspector is a serious offence.) An inspector has the following powers:

(a) To enter premises and, if resisted, to obtain the support of a police officer.

(b) To inspect premises.

(c) To require that evidence, etc is not disturbed following an incident.

(d) To take measurements and photographs, although it is usual to ask permission in the latter case.

(e) To take samples of suspect substances.

(f) To require tests to be carried out on suspect substances or equipment.

(g) To require plant or equipment to be dismantled.

(h) To require anyone who has knowledge relevant to the matter being investigated to give it either verbally or in writing. (The inspector has discretion to permit another person to be present during questioning or the taking of a written statement. The person making a written statement is required to sign it and it is an offence to make a false statement in these circumstances. Any information given by a person to an inspector prior to a formal caution ("you are not obliged to say anything, but anything you say may be used in evidence against you") cannot be used in criminal proceedings against that person.

(i) To inspect and take copies of statutory records and other relevant documents.

(j) To require assistance from anyone within that person's limits of responsibilities. (It is an offence to obstruct an inspector.)

(k) To issue improvement and prohibition notices.

(l) To recommend that prosecutions are brought.

Notices

Where a breach of law has occurred, or is likely to occur, inspectors can issue improvement notices. An improvement notice must state what the legal breach is believed to be and the reason for that belief. It should also specify a time limit in which the matter in question must be rectified.

If any situation is found that is such as to constitute an immediate risk of serious personal injury an inspector may issue a prohibition notice, which requires that the activity in question is stopped pending the taking of remedial action. There does not have to be a specific breach of the law. The notice must detail the matters which, in the inspector's opinion, give rise to the risk. If the risk is not immediate a deferred prohibition notice can be issued, giving a date after which the activity must cease unless the remedial work has been carried out. Where, despite every effort being made, it has not proved possible to meet such a deadline, inspectors may be prepared to extend the deferment period. Requests for this must, however, be made before the notice has expired.

Inspectors will usually discuss the terms of any notice with the head-teacher and other interested parties such as safety representatives. They will endeavour to specify a reasonable time for rectification, taking into account considerations like examinations, the time needed to obtain new equipment and, sometimes, the availability of funds.

If there are changes in circumstances which make the original notice inappropriate before the end of the specified period, the inspector should be advised. The inspector can withdraw or amend a notice in such cases.

It is possible to appeal against a notice to an industrial tribunal within 21 days of the notice being served. Improvement notices are suspended until the appeal is decided but prohibition notices remain in force unless the tribunal agrees to an application for suspension.

A notice is a legal sanction and prosecution is likely to follow in any case where it is found that its requirements have been disregarded.

Enforcement in schools

It can be seen that the law provides inspectors with considerable powers to assist them in carrying out their enforcement role. In practice, however, they apply those powers sparingly, generally preferring to pursue compliance in a courteous, sensitive manner. This is sometimes misunderstood and when, for example, inspectors prefer politely to make appointments rather than walk into schools unannounced, they should not be left sitting outside the head's study for half an hour!

Inspectors aim to achieve a situation where every school and LEA has effective management arrangements and procedures to deal with problems without their becoming involved. If, for example, safety representatives seek the assistance of inspectors the response will normally be to enquire whether management has been given the opportunity to achieve a solution.

If existing channels have not been explored a safety representative will probably be referred back to management in the first instance. (Some trade unions recommend that their safety representatives should, whenever possible, consult headquarters before contacting the HSE.)

Inspectors may visit schools in response to information provided to them about specific problems, to investigate incidents or, on a routine basis, to look at health and safety standards either generally or in certain areas.

If inspectors find matters requiring rectification they have various options open to them. They may decide to give written or verbal advice, they may provide relevant information in the form of advisory leaflets, etc, they may issue notices or they may consider legal proceedings. The procedure adopted will depend on various factors, such as how blatant the breach of the law is, what the general standards of health and safety in the school are, whether the school has a satisfactory written statement of arrangements, whether the matter has been raised before, and the attitude of the people involved towards health and safety. The inspector will certainly seek to ensure that any action taken will result in the correction of any immediate problems and make any similar occurrence extremely unlikely.

The power to prosecute is also used sparingly. Depending on the circumstances, the employer (eg the LEA or governors in a voluntary aided school), the individual members of staff or both may be taken to court. The inspector, having collected evidence (eg by taking statements or collecting samples) and having decided that a prosecution may be warranted, prepares a prosecution report. This states the case for court action, the reasons for recommending prosecution and any mitigating circumstances. If the case is approved by the inspectors' line manager, a summons is issued. In England and Wales accused persons have, for most cases, the option of electing to appear before the magistrates' court where the maximum fine is £20,000 for each breach of ss.2 to 6 HASAWA (up to £5000 for breaches of regulations), or to go to trial in a higher court. On indictment unlimited fines can be imposed and, for offences such as breaching a prohibition notice, individuals may be sentenced to a term of imprisonment.

The vast majority of inspectors are highly professional, very knowledgeable and do not try to exceed their authority. Cases of an inspector falling below this standard are almost unheard of, but if such a problem should arise, the inspector should be asked for the name of his or her senior officer who should be contacted to discuss the matter.

Information for Employees

The Health and Safety (Information for Employees) Regulations 1989 were made under HASAWA. They require that employees are given basic information about health and safety law and the address of the local office of the enforcing authority and of the Health and Safety Executive's Employment Medical Advisory Service.

Requirements under legislation such as the Factories Act 1961 and the Offices, Shops and Railway Premises Act 1963 to display abstracts of the law relevant to such workplaces were repealed by these regulations.

There are two simple methods available to employers to meet these requirements. The HSE has approved a poster and a leaflet, copies of which are available from HMSO. If the leaflet option is chosen, arrangements must be made to ensure that all future new employees are also provided with a copy. The posters are A2 size, encapsulated in plastic with spaces for the appropriate addresses to be added. Compliance with the regulations will be achieved if one or more posters are displayed so that all employees have the opportunity to read them.

Addresses of HSC and HSE Offices, etc

Health and Safety Commission: Baynards House, 1 Chepstow Place, Westbourne Grove, London W2 4TF

HSE Education National Interest Group and *Education Service Advisory Committee*: Maritime House, 1 Linton Road, Barking, Essex IG11 8HF (081-594 5522)

HSE Information Services: Broad Lane, Sheffield S3 7HQ (0742 892345) (Fax 0742 892333).

HSE Freeleaflet Line Service: 0742 892346

Employment Medical Advisory Service. Baynards House, 1 Chepstow Place, Westbourne Grove, London W2 4TF.

HSE area offices

East Anglia: (Essex, Norfolk and Suffolk) 39 Baddow Road, Chelmsford, Essex CM2 0HL (0245 284661).

Northern Home Counties: (Bedfordshire, Buckinghamshire, Cambridgeshire, Hertfordshire) 14 Cardiff Road, Luton, Beds LU1 1PP (0582 34121).

East Midlands: (Leicestershire, Northamptonshire, Oxfordshire, Warwickshire) Belgrave House, 1 Greyfriars, Northampton NN1 2BS (0604 21233).

West Midlands: McLaren Buildings, 2 Masshouse Circus, Queensway, Birmingham B4 7NP (021-200 2299).

Wales: (Clwyd, Dyfed, Gwent, Gwynedd, Mid Glamorgan, Powys, South Glamorgan, West Glamorgan) Brunel House, 2 Fitzalan Road, Cardiff CF2 1SH (0222 473777).

The Marches: (Hereford, Worcester, Shropshire, Staffordshire) The Marches House, Midway, Newcastle under Lyme, Staffs ST5 1DT (0782 717181).

North Midlands: (Derbyshire, Lincolnshire, Nottinghamshire) Birbeck House, Trinity Square, Nottingham NG1 4AU (0602 470712).

South West: (Avon, Cornwall, Devon, Gloucestershire, Somerset, Isles of Scilly) Inter City House, Mitchell Lane, Victoria Street, Bristol BS1 6AN (0272 290681).

South: (Berkshire, Dorset, Hampshire, Isle of Wight, Wiltshire) Priestley House, Priestley Road, Basingstoke RG24 9NW (0256 473181).

South East: (Kent, Surrey, East Sussex, West Sussex) 3 East Grinstead House, London Road, East Grinstead, Sussex RH19 1RR (0342 26922).

London North: (Barking and Dagenham, Barnet, Brent, Camden, Ealing, Enfield, Hackney, Haringey, Harrow, Havering, Islington, Newham, Redbridge, Tower Hamlets, Waltham Forest) Maritime House, 1 Linton Road, Barking, Essex IG11 8HF (081-594 5522) and Chancel House, Neasden Lane, London NW10 2UD (081-459 8855).

London South: (Bexley, Bromley, City of London, Croydon, Greenwich, Hammersmith and Fulham, Hillingdon, Hounslow, Kensington and Chelsea, Kingston, Lambeth, Lewisham, Merton, Richmond, Southwark, Sutton, Wandsworth, Westminster) 1 Long Lane, London SE1 4PG (071-407 8911).

South Yorkshire: (Humberside, South Yorkshire) Sovereign House, 40 Silver Street, Sheffield S1 2ES (0742 739081).

West and North Yorkshire: 8 St Paul's Street, Leeds LS1 2LE (0532 446191).

Greater Manchester: Quay House, Quay Street, Manchester M3 3JB (061-831 7111).

Merseyside: (Cheshire, Merseyside) The Triad, Stanley Road, Bootle, Merseyside L20 3PG (051-922 7211).

North West: (Cumbria, Lancashire) Victoria House, Ormskirk Road, Preston PR1 1HH (0772 59321).

North East: (Cleveland, Durham, Northumberland, Tyne and Wear) Arden House, Regent Centre, Regent Farm Road, Gosforth, Newcastle upon Tyne NE3 3JN (091-284 8448).

Scotland East: (Borders, Central, Fife, Grampian, Highland, Lothian, Tayside, Orkney and Shetland) Belford House, 59 Belford Road, Edinburgh EH4 3UE (031-225 1313).

Scotland West: (Dumfries and Galloway, Strathclyde and the Western Isles) Royal Exchange Assurance House, 314 St Vincent Street, Glasgow G3 8XG (041-204 2646) and Lord Cullen House, Fraser Place, Aberdeen AB9 1UB (0224 252500).

Chapter 3
Management of Health and Safety

The responsibilities of schools' managements in respect of health and safety date back to the day that the first school opened its doors. Schools have always had rules and arrangements designed to avoid and deal with problems. The ethos of schools was such that in the past many arrangements were *ad hoc*, relying on the goodwill and the commitment of staff, rather than formalised systems. The introduction of the Health and Safety at Work, etc Act 1974 (HASAWA), however, made explicit requirements that previously had been implicit. Health and safety now had to be formally managed, and managed effectively.

In the 1970s many headteachers would have been offended to have been described as managers, even though this aspect of their role was spelled out clearly in the Articles of Government. Given local management of schools (LMS) it is difficult to believe that in 1978 one large education authority and its headteachers indulged in a long formal dispute as to whether heads were managers of schools. It was also indicative of the difficulties of introducing into education the type of management previously found only in business and commerce that the Education Officer of that authority found it necessary to write to schools to say that when he requested that something be done, he required that it be done.

Health and safety is not a separate entity. It is an integral part of the management of schools and its implications need to be considered to an appropriate degree whenever decisions are made. There are three primary reasons why this must be so.

Humanitarian Reasons for "Health and Safety"

Personal injury can have a severe and lasting effect on the victim, while a premature death can scar the lives of both relatives and those who feel responsible for it. An accident may result in a lifetime of pain, being unable to continue with a career, and/or being forced to endure a permanent reduction of the quality of life. We have a moral duty to each other that requires that we take all reasonable measures to try to avoid such occurrences.

Legal Reasons for "Health and Safety"

The law requires that due regard is paid to health and safety and can apply significant sanctions on organisations and individuals who are negligent in this respect. Prior to 1975 injuries arising from negligence may have resulted in a civil action, with the insurance company being the loser, but HASAWA is criminal legislation and it is not possible to insure against fines and imprisonment, or against the implications of having had a criminal conviction.

Economic Reasons for "Health and Safety"

The introduction of LMS has transferred the impact of the uninsured costs of accidents from LEAs to schools. Accidents have always cost money, but in the past such costs have been lost in centralised budgets. Generous staffing levels often meant that absences could be absorbed with little more than inconvenience. Circumstances have now changed and accidents could prove to be a significant drain on local staffing and maintenance budgets. The uninsured losses arising from an accident may include:

(a) the cost of the lost time of the injured person
(b) the cost of a temporary replacement member of staff
(c) the cost of repairs to the premises, equipment, plant, etc
(d) the cost of management and administrative time absorbed by investigations, reporting, etc
(e) the loss to the education process caused by the absence of staff or the non-availability of equipment, etc awaiting repair.

Even if staff are able to cover for an absent colleague for a day or two there will be a loss of efficiency unless more staff are being employed than are actually needed.

It is comparatively easy to calculate the loss arising when a teacher slips on a newly washed floor, breaks a leg and is absent for a term. It is not possible objectively to measure the effects of bad publicity arising from, say, the death of a pupil or a prosecution.

Responsibility and Delegation

The extent to which anyone is responsible for health and safety matters is effectively limited by his or her contract of employment. It is only possible to have responsibility for those matters over which one has executive authority. Parliament, in making legislation, often incorporates new implied terms into employees' contracts but these are still subject to the same principle. Headteachers are responsible for everything over which they have control, and where they do not have such control (eg over capital expenditure needed to eliminate a hazard) they are expected to take all reasonable measures within their executive authority to avoid or minimise the problem. A head of department (HOD) is responsible for health and safety within the department, while class teachers are responsible for the immediate area of their work. Again, if class teachers discover a hazard the law requires them to take all reasonable steps within their executive authority to eliminate it and to refer the matter to their HOD or headteacher if the limits of their authority preclude a permanent solution (for example, if a hole is found in the corridor the class teacher will be expected to take all reasonable measures to stop anyone falling into it pending a decision by the headteacher to close the area).

Those who have a responsibility can delegate the tasks necessary to discharge it but they cannot delegate the responsibility itself. If tasks are delegated there is a very clear incentive for the person whose neck remains on the block to monitor effectively the way that the tasks are being carried out. The headteacher who passes "responsibility" for health and safety to a junior member of staff and then puts it out of mind could be likened to the person who jumped off a tall building and remarked, on passing the third floor window, that it was all right so far.

Governors

The various changes in the management and control of schools over recent years has caused doubts about the extent to which school governors are responsible in law for their actions. The position in this respect is in fact very simple. Whatever the particular status of their school, governors are responsible to the limit of their executive powers. If, for example, there is a legal requirement for training but an LMS governing body with delegated control of the training budget decides not to fund an appropriate course they are liable to prosecution. If, however, the allocated budget is inadequate they will have discharged their legal responsibilities if they formally bring the shortfall to the attention of the LEA and instruct the headteacher to take any necessary measures to avoid possible consequential breaches of the law (eg untrained staff to be instructed not to use woodworking machines).

Whilst in county and controlled schools in England and Wales the LEA remains the employer of school staff, governors have some degree of control of the school premises. S. 4 Health and Safety at Work, etc Act requires that persons with control of premises take measures to ensure, so far as is reasonably practicable, that the premises, equipment and substances used there are safe and without risk to health. In non LMS county schools the governors will have little such control compared to those in LMS establishments, and in the first case they may need simply to bring a matter to the attention of the LEA, while in the second they may need to allocate funds.

It is most important that governors are fully aware of the extent of the control of premises, budgets, etc that has been delegated to them, and should ask for written clarification of any such areas that are not clear to them.

Statement of Health and Safety Policy and Arrangements

The key to the effective management of health and safety in a school is the statement of policy and arrangements. Every employer with more than five employees is required (by s.2 HASAWA) to produce and to keep under review such a statement. It must be brought to the attention of all employees.

The statement should consist of three parts. Part 1 should be a statement of the employer's policy and attitude towards health and safety. This should be written by, or on behalf of, the leader of the LEA, the chair of governors, etc. Part 2 should detail the organisation intended to carry out that policy. It should spell out the responsibilities and tasks of managers and employees, how safety representatives and safety committees are involved, and how implementation of the policy is to be monitored. Part 3 should describe the arrangements established to cover such matters as inspections, first aid, fire precautions, etc. The statement should be such as to ensure that all employees know what is expected of them and what they need to do to discharge their legal responsibilities.

LEAs obviously cannot issue a single document describing on one hand the philosophy and policy of the elected members and on the other detail such as who is responsible for maintaining the contents of the first aid box in every school. It is the usual practice for LEAs to publish a statement of policy, together with the service-wide organisation and arrangements. Each school is instructed to produce a statement covering the local organisation and arrangements which is then attached to the LEA document to form a complete response to the s.2 HASAWA requirement.

Voluntary aided and independent schools will be able to produce a single statement containing all the necessary elements. Reading statements prepared for and by various schools it is apparent that there remains some reticence on the part of governors, LEAs, etc when it comes to spelling out requirements. Headteachers and staff are still being requested rather than instructed to carry out responsibilities and tasks. Such niceties are misleading and are likely to be misunderstood by Health and Safety Executive (HSE) inspectors and the courts.

Part 1—Statement of policy and intent

The following is an example of what might be issued by a LEA.

(a) The Members of Loamshire County Council consider that one of their primary objectives is the achievement and maintenance of a high standard of health and safety on all its premises.

(b) They also recognise and accept their corporate responsibility to provide a healthy and safe working environment for all their employees and for members of the public using Council premises.

(c) They will take all reasonably practicable steps to fulfil this responsibility and will pay particular attention to meeting the requirements of the Health and Safety at Work, etc Act 1974 and all relevant statutory provisions.

(d) They require management at all levels to display a positive attitude towards health and safety.

(e) The Members require employees at all levels to pursue the Council's objectives in respect of health and safety.

(f) The Council will employ professionally qualified safety advisors to advise on the effective implementaton of its policies and objectives.

(g) It will maintain arrangements with staff trade unions for joint consultation on and participation in measures for promoting health and safety.

(h) The Education Officer will ensure that a suitable organisation is set up and arrangements are maintained to carry out the Council's requirements in respect of the Education Department and all education establishments.

Signed A SMITH
Chairman

Governors of voluntary aided and independent schools can adapt the above example to suit their circumstances. Some voluntary aided schools, however, elect to tie themselves into the LEA's arrangements, but this does not absolve the governors of their responsibility to produce a statement, such as:

(a) The governors of St Mary's RC Junior School recognise their corporate responsibility as an employer to provide a safe and healthy environment for the teaching and non-teaching staff, the pupils and other people who come onto the premises.

(b) They will take all reasonably practicable steps within their power to fulfil this responsibility.

(c) It is the intention of the governors that for health and safety purposes the school will operate within the structure and framework of Loamshire County Council and will apply all health and safety instructions and advice issued by the Education Department as if St Mary's were a maintained school.

(d) The headteacher is required to draw up the necessary arrangements to secure compliance with all health and safety requirements, to write them down and to circulate this information to all staff and to ourselves, and subsequently to monitor implementation of the arrangements.

Signed A BROWN
Chairman of Governors

Part 2—Description of organisation

The need for a separate "Part 2" in large organisations is explained above. It should spell out the duties and responsibilities of the various managers involved. These may include the personnel officer, the council architect, the engineer, the council's safety advisor and, depending on the organisation, senior officers in charge of catering, transport, etc.

Most importantly of all, it should spell out in detail what is expected of headteachers. Typically a headteacher will be directed:

(a) To pursue the objectives of the Council in respect of health and safety.

(b) To set up arrangements in the school to cover all health and safety legal requirements, to produce a written statement of those arrangements, and to bring it, and Parts 1 and 2 of the Council's statement, to the attention of all staff. The statement is to be revised and republished as necessary. To monitor effectively the implementation of the arrangements.

(c) To be available to any member of staff to discuss and to seek to resolve health and safety problems not solved at a lower level or through the established arrangements.

(d) To report to the education department those instances where the head's executive authority does not allow the elimination or reduction to a satisfactory level of a hazard, but to take all necessary short term measures to avoid danger pending rectification.

(e) To note all health and safety instructions and advice issued by the Council and to ensure that they are brought to the attention of all staff. To keep a file of such information together with information and advice published by the DES and others about the health and safety aspects of the activities carried on in the school, and to make this information available to all staff.

(f) To keep a list of safety representatives appointed to represent staff at the school, to be readily available to them, and to cooperate with them as far as is reasonable in their efforts to carry out their functions. To receive written reports from safety representatives and to respond in writing within a reasonable time.

(g) To establish a school safety committee within three months of receiving a written request from two safety representatives of staff at the school.

(h) To ensure that all areas of the school are inspected once per term.

(i) To ensure that a system is established for the reporting, recording and investigation of accidents, and that all reasonable steps are taken to prevent recurrences.

(j) To ensure that all visitors, including maintenance contractors, are informed of any hazards on site of which they may be unaware. To ensure that consideration is given to the possibilities of maintenance work affecting pupils and staff.

(k) To ensure that new employees are briefed about safety arrangements; in particular to ensure they are given a copy of the school's statement and the opportunity to read it before starting work.

(l) To ensure the use of any necessary protective clothing and equipment, and that it is properly maintained and renewed when required.

(m) To ensure that effective arrangements are in force to facilitate ready evacuation of the buildings in case of fire or other emergency, and that fire fighting equipment is available and maintained.

Part 3—The school's arrangements

This statement is primarily intended to inform all staff of the ways and means by which the headteacher intends to meet the various requirements of legislation. It should spell out to staff what is expected of them and what they should do in foreseeable emergency situations. In the event of a visit from a Health and Safety Executive inspector it will also indicate the general approach of the management to health and safety and pinpoint where the blame lies in any breakdown in arrangements. In secondary schools heads of departments such as science, CDT, art and home economics should be instructed to draw up written statements of arrangements covering the special needs of their areas. These should be appended to the general school statement.

The school statement should cover the following matters:

(a) Accidents (who is to be informed, who is responsible for statutory notification, how details are to be recorded, who carries out any investigation). (See "Accidents".)

(b) First aid (who is responsible for giving first aid, where first aid boxes are located and who is responsible for maintaining them, who summons an ambulance, accompanies pupils to hospital, informs parents, governors, etc). (See "First Aid".)

(c) Fire precautions (frequency of drills, procedures to be followed, maintenance of exits and escape routes; who is responsible for ensuring that extinguishers, etc are maintained; who summons the fire brigade). (See "Fire".)

(d) Hazards (everyone responsible for identification, who hazards should be reported to, interim measures to be taken pending rectification, who is responsible for arranging for remedial works).

(e) Environment (how defects in heating, lighting, ventilation, etc are to be reported and who is responsible for progressing repairs).

(f) Safety representatives and safety committee (who the safety representatives are, the structure and membership of the school committee and the means by which staff can have issues raised there). (See "Safety Representatives and Safety Committees".)

(g) Inspections (who will carry them out, how frequent, etc). (See "Inspections" and "Engineering Inspections".)

(h) Information (details of where staff can obtain advice and information about the health and safety implications of their activities, and about substances and articles used at school). (See "Information".)

(i) Substances (how the introduction of new substances is to be controlled, storage of flammable liquids, etc). (See "Control of substances hazardous to health", "Storage of Hazardous Substances".)

(j) New staff (how, when and by whom they will be briefed about the school's arrangements).

(k) Electrical safety (inspection of equipment by users and periodically by "competent persons", any limitations on bringing personal items to school, etc). (See "Electrical Safety".)

(l) Infectious diseases (how staff will be informed of any cases, necessary precautions, etc). (See "Infectious diseases".)

In addition to the above, details should be included of any arrangements that are necessary to cover unusual local conditions (eg premises shared with others).

The statement should spell out the legal responsibilities imposed on all staff by s.7 and s.8 HASAWA. (See "The law and related issues—Health and Safety at Work, etc Act".)

Monitoring

When the statement is drawn up any safety representatives appointed to cover staff at the school should be consulted on its content. It should be brought to the attention of all staff, teaching and non-teaching, and implemented. Periodic checks and routine inspections of the premises should be made to ensure that the stated arrangements are in force and are effective.

A school and a local authority were recently prosecuted following the death by drowning of a pupil on a sponsored swim at a local swimming pool. He was one of a party of ten handicapped pupils supervised by five members of staff from the school, none of whom had recent life saving qualifications and none of whom was formally in charge. The local authority had written to swimming clubs shortly before the accident saying that bookings would be accepted subject to qualified lifeguards being on hand. The school, however, was unaware of this requirement while the lifeguard and manager employed at the pool by the local authority believed that the school staff were providing expert supervision for the pupils. The local authority was fined £2500 with £7000 costs, while the school was fined £500 with £1000 costs. During the trial the arrangements were described as "sloppy" and afterwards the HSE inspector who brought the case spoke of the need for positive acts by managers. "This", he said "includes tight and effective supervision so that when instructions are issued they are actually put into practice. It is not acceptable to issue instructions and subsequently to take no further action."

Advice

It is important that headteachers identify sources of expert advice and use them when in any doubt. LEAs may well employ safety advisors who are trained in all aspects of occupational health and safety. The local authority will employ environmental health officers who will be able to give advice on matters such as pest control, water quality and food hygiene. The school doctor and the senior nursing officer of the local district health authority will be able to provide assistance on matters relating to infectious diseases, administration of medicines to pupils, head lice, etc. Health and Safety Executive inspectors, at the local area office, are usually willing to give advice on matters relating to health and safety law and its application to schools, and if they are unable to assist they may well be able to advise where help can be obtained.

Consultants

Much recent legislation will require school employers who do not have access to in-house expertise to obtain such help externally. Whilst schools do have the option of sending a member of staff for specific training to meet this need such a course is unlikely to be cost effective except in the case of large multi-school organisations.

The Approved Code of Practice accompanying the Management of Health and Safety at Work Regulations (MHSWR) states that employers are "solely responsible" for ensuring that consultants are competent to carry out the assigned tasks. It is therefore unfortunate, to say the least, that at the time of writing there is no national agreement on the minimum level of professional training and experience necessary for persons offering their services as health and safety consultants. Government ministers and the Health and Safety Executive (HSE) have recently severely criticised the activities of incompetent and/or avaricious individuals and organisations operating in this field. Cases have occurred where HSE Inspectors have needed to issue enforcement notices to correct errors made by such consultants. Schools have been involved in considerable and unnecessary expense when they have accepted advice to install systems appropriate to deal with the hazards of a factory production line rather than the occasional, small scale use of equipment in CDT workshops.

While the majority of consultants will do a professional job and provide good value for money the problem of identifying those who are honest, competent and have a proper appreciation of the nature of schools and their work can be daunting. It is recommended that where the services of safety advisors working for the local education authority (LEA) are available they should be purchased as necessary. If this is not an option the local HSE area office or the LEA safety advisor may be able to recommend a competent consultant with experience in the field of education. If all else fails, and it proves necessary to buy a "pig in a poke", it is suggested that at least two written quotations are obtained and the advice of the local HSE Inspector is sought about any obviously dubious points before a decision is made.

Employers are required to consult with safety representatives "in good time" with regard to the arrangements for the appointment of a consultant to meet the requirements of the MHSWR (see "Consultation, facilities and assistance, Safety Representatives and Safety Committees").

When briefing a consultant to carry out an assessment of a school to meet the requirements of Regulation 3 MHSWR it should be remembered that other more specific assessments are required by recent legislation. It is sensible to engage a consultant who is able and willing to carry out all immediately necessary assessment work required by:

(a) the Management of Health and Safety at Work Regulations 1992
(b) the Provision and Use of Work Equipment Regulations 1992
(c) the Personal Protective Equipment at Work Regulations 1992
(d) the Health and Safety (Display Screen Equipment) Regulations 1992
(e) the Manual Handling Operations Regulations 1992
(f) the Control of Substances Hazardous to Health Regulations 1988.

(This last mentioned requirement should only involve checking in place arrangements for compliance.)

It is suggested that a consultant also be asked to prepare a separate report detailing those alterations to premises required to be made by 1 January 1996 to achieve compliance with the Workplace (Health, Safety and Welfare) Regulations 1992.

The HSE has published a free leaflet which gives general guidance on choosing a consultant.

Further reading

Safety Polices in the Educational Sector, HMSO 1985
Writing your health and safety policy statement: how to prepare a statement for a small business (rev.), HMSO 1989
Successful health and safety management, HMSO 1991
The School Governor's Legal Guide, 5th edition, Croner 1990
Responsibilities of school governors for health and safety, HMSO 1992
Selecting a Health and Safety Consultancy IND(G) 133L, HSE 1992

Chapter 4

Management of Health and Safety at Work Regulations 1992

The Management of Health and Safety at Work Regulations 1992 spell out in more detail how compliance with the general duties laid down in the parent legislation (Health and Safety at Work, etc Act) is to be achieved. They have been framed to cover workplaces from major chemical plants to nursery schools. Those requirements which have no relevance to schools have been disregarded. When considering the application of these regulations to schools it must be borne in mind that the "employer" requirements are perforce subject to the same limits of reasonable practicability as the parent legislation.

Risk Assessment

Regulation 3 requires employers to carry out an assessment of the risks to the health and safety of staff while at work, and that of others arising from the conduct of the undertaking. The assessment should identify those measures which must be taken to ensure compliance with all relevant health and safety legislation. An assessment must be reviewed (and amended if necessary) when there is reason to suppose that it is no longer valid or there has been a significant change in an area in question. Where the employer employs more than five persons the significant findings of the assessment and details of any employees identified as being especially at risk must be formally recorded. Most schools already carry out informal risk assessments on a day to day basis. This regulation, however, places an absolute duty on employers to carry out a formal, systematic examination of the premises, equipment and work activities, and to write down all significant matters identified by that examination. Significant matters will include:

(a) non-compliance with relevant specific legislation
(b) hazards not covered by specific legislation but where the risk has not been controlled so far as is reasonably practicable (see appendix)
(c) requirements for training not covered by specific legislation but needed to comply with Regulation 11 and/or s.2 Health and Safety at Work, etc Act
(d) identification of needs for more detailed assessment work, etc required by other health and safety legislation.

(Detailed information on the carrying out of assessments is given in the Approved Code of Practice (ACOP).)

All foreseeable risks should be considered although trivial risks may be disregarded.

Employers are required by Regulation 6 to appoint "one or more" competent persons to assist in achieving compliance with all statutory health and safety requirements. The time and means at the disposal of "competent persons" must be adequate to carry out their tasks, taking account of the nature and size of the undertaking. Where the appointed person is not an employee the employer must provide him or her with all information about known or suspected factors affecting the health and safety of employees or others using the site. A "competent person" is one who "has had sufficient training and experience or knowledge and other qualities to enable him/her properly to assist in undertaking the measures referred to". (In county and controlled schools the employer is the LEA, and most LEAs will already have safety officers or advisors to carry out this role. Where this is not the case, and where other types of school are concerned, the choice will be between nominating a member of staff and providing them with appropriate training, or buying in the services of a consultant. (See "Consultants").)

Regulation 3 requires employers to have arrangements in place to cover health and safety which are appropriate for the size and nature of the undertaking. (See "Statement of Health and Safety Policy and Arrangements". The Approved Code of Practice (ACOP) specifies that details of the "competent person" appointed under Regulation 6 should be appended to the health and safety policy statement, together with the report of significant findings arising from the assessment demanded by Regulation 3.)

Health Surveillance

Where the assessment identifies risks to health which warrant formal health surveillance, Regulation 5 requires the employer to provide it. The ACOP lays down strict criteria which almost certainly rule out such a requirement for staff in schools. It is possible that some consultants may consider that cleaning and/or catering staff require surveillance to detect early signs of dermatitis (see "Dermatitis").

Evacuation of Premises

Regulation 7 is concerned with the emergency evacuation of workplaces in the event of "serious and imminent danger". It relates to schools in that there must be appropriate procedures in place to allow for efficient evacuation of the premises in the event of fire, bomb threats, etc (see "Fire").

Information

Regulation 8 requires an employer to provide employees with information about risks to their health and safety that have been identified by the assessment, and about the preventative and protective measures required to counter those risks. Employees must also be given details about the evacuation procedures required by Regulation 7, and about risks to their safety and health notified to the employer by other employers working on the same site. The ACOP limits the extent of the information that must be provided about risks and precautions to that which the employees need to know to ensure their health and safety. Information must be capable of being understood by the employees, with due regard being given to the needs of persons with disabilities or language difficulties.

Information from "other employers" (see Regulation 9, below) may arise where premises are shared with other establishments or where contractors are working at the school.

Where persons such as contractor's employees or temporary workers are working on another employer's premises Regulation 10 requires that they and their employer are provided by the occupier with comprehensible information about any risks to their health and safety arising from the conduct of the occupier's undertaking, and details of any legally required measures taken in respect of the health and safety of such workers or employees. The occupier must also ensure that such workers and their employers are informed about emergency evacuation procedures.

Where schools are concerned, contractor's employees carrying out cleaning, repairs, installations and maintenance are likely to be specialists in their fields and better informed than the school of the risks of their respective occupations. The information provided by the school should be concerned with those risks which are peculiar to the premises or the school's activities (eg the provisions made to enable windows to be cleaned safely, the implications of class change signals for a contractor using a ladder in a corridor or an outbreak of bacillary dysentery).

Temporary staff hired from an agency must be properly briefed when first starting work. Where the school has a comprehensive health and safety statement (see "Statement of Health and Safety Policy and arrangements") its provision, the time to read it, and a check to ensure that it is understood, will meet this statutory requirement.

Where LEA staff work in hospitals, Department of Social Security premises, etc they and the LEA must be given similar information by the employer responsible for the premises.

Regulation 13 deals with the need to provide information to persons employed on fixed-duration contracts or who are employed by an agency but are working under the control of a "user". Before employees on fixed-duration contracts start work they must be informed of any special occupational qualifications or skills required to enable the work to be carried out safely and be given details of any legally required health surveillance to which they will be subject. Agency workers must be given similar information. Users of agency workers must inform the agency employer of the above skills requirements and any "specific features" of the post to be filled which might affect their health and safety. The agency employer must pass this information to employees. ("Specific features" might include the need to lift pupils with disabilities or deal with pupils with serious behavioural problems.)

Cooperation and Coordination

Where two or more employers share a workplace, even when this is not on a permanent basis, Regulation 9 requires them to cooperate as necessary to enable compliance with health and safety law. They must coordinate the measures each takes to meet statutory health and safety requirements, and take all reasonable steps to inform each other of any risks to health and safety arising from work activities, etc which might affect the other's employees. A self-employed person is considered "an employer" in this respect.

This regulation will mainly apply to schools when contractors are carrying out work on the premises. (Although school premises are often used by other organisations, such as adult evening institutes, both users usually have the same employer and this regulation will not apply. However, although not a specific requirement under this regulation, cooperation and coordination of health and safety measures between such site users will be needed to meet the general requirements of the Health and Safety at Work, etc Act). (See "Contractors on School Premises".)

Capabilities and Training

Regulation 11 requires employers, when entrusting tasks to employees, to take into account their capabilities as regards health and safety. Employees must receive adequate health and safety training when first recruited, and when being exposed to new or additional risks because of a change of work, the need to use new or different work equipment, or the introduction of new technology or changed systems of working. This training must be repeated as necessary, be adapted so as to remain relevant to the health and safety risks in question and take place in working hours.

Employers are required to ensure that tasks allocated to employees do not exceed their ability to carry them out without risk to themselves or others. When making such a judgement the employer is expected to give due regard to the employee's capabilities, training, knowledge and experience. All staff should receive induction training in health and safety, and in schools this should be based on the arrangements for first aid, fire drill procedures, sources of information, etc, as spelled out in the statement of policy and arrangements. In most schools it is the blue collar areas where training is most needed and least often carried out. Bringing up a family is not adequate training for work in a school kitchen, or using commercial cleaning and food preparation machines (see "School Kitchens"). Additional training needs should be identified by the risk assessment carried out under Regulation 3. The advice of the person making the assessment should be sought on the scale and content of any recommended training.

Employee's Duties

Employees are required to use any "machinery, equipment, dangerous substance, transport equipment, means of production or safety device" provided by the employer in accordance with any training received from, and instructions given by, the employer which are in compliance with health and safety law. Regulation 12 also requires employees to inform the employer of any work situation which persons of their training and instruction would reasonably consider represented a serious and immediate danger to health and safety, or a shortcoming in the employer's protective arrangements. These latter requirements are subject to the proviso that the situation or shortcoming either affects the health and safety of the employee in question, or arises out of or in connection with the employee's work activities, and has not been previously reported.

This regulation emphasises the nature of the duty placed on employees by s.7 Health and Safety at Work, etc Act which requires them to take reasonable care of themselves and of others who may be affected by their acts and omissions in the workplace. The second duty under s.7 requires cooperation with employers so that they comply with their statutory duties, hence the duty to report dangerous situations and shortcomings in arrangements.

Civil Liability

Regulation 15 states that a breach of these regulations does not constitute a breach of statutory duty in a civil law sense. (This has been included because the wording of most of the regulations is too generalised to allow a virtually automatic award of damages on proving a breach of any one of them. This would not preclude a claim for compensation for injuries arising from such a breach but other grounds, such as negligence, would have to be proved (see "Insurance and Compensation").)

Regulation 17 amends the Safety Representatives and Safety Committee

Regulations 1977 by adding an additional Regulation, 4A (see "Safety Representatives and Safety Committees").

Further reading

Managment of Health and Safety at Work (Regulations and Approved Code of Practice), HSC 1992, HMSO

Chapter 5

Safety Representatives and Safety Committees

The Robens Report said that the promotion of health and safety at work is first and foremost a matter of efficient management, but that it is not a management prerogative. S.2 of the Health and Safety at Work, etc Act 1974 (HASAWA) was drafted with the need to involve all employees in mind. By s.2(4) the Act recognised that trade unions were given the right to appoint safety representatives at places of work. S.2(6) states that representatives must be consulted by employers with a view to the making and maintenance of arrangements which will enable effective cooperation in achieving safe conditions of work. The employer is required to establish a safety committee to monitor safety matters if the representatives so wish (s.2(7)).

Originally, under s.2(5), employees at workplaces where unions are not recognised were able to elect safety representatives. This subsection was deleted by the Employment Protection Act 1975, leaving a situation where only trade unions can make such appointments. This effectively meant that about half the total workforce lost the legal right to be consulted on safety matters and to have safety committees.

The s.2 requirements were subsequently supplemented by the Safety Representatives and Safety Committee Regulations 1977, which were accompanied by an approved code of practice and guidance notes. A further approved code of practice (HSC 9), covering time off for training, was published in 1978.

The Regulations and Codes of Practice

The regulations, the two approved codes of practice and the guidance notes are now published in a single booklet. The preface says that the Health and Safety Commission views the regulations and codes of practice as providing "a legal framework within which employers and trade unions can make arrangements for the functioning of safety committees and safety representatives". The regulations do not attempt to lay down a ratio of safety representatives to employees or the method of selection to be used where a number of trade unions have members at a workplace. These and similar questions are left to agreement between the employer and the trade unions, and between the trade unions. The preface also says that employers and employees may draw up alternative arrangements for joint consultation over health and safety that do not follow the provisions and advice given in the booklet but that trade unions can invoke the rights provided by the regulations at any time they choose to do so.

Safety Representatives

Appointment of safety representatives

A recognised trade union may appoint safety representatives at a workplace where it has one or more members. A "recognised trade union" broadly means an independent trade union recognised by the employer for pay negotiation purposes. The trade union must advise the employer in writing of the appointment, and state the group of staff to be represented. Persons appointed should, so far as is reasonably practicable, have worked for the employer for the previous two years or have had at least two years' experience in similar employment.

It is not unusual for six or more trade unions to have members among staff in a nursery school, and in secondary schools there may be as many as a dozen unions who could appoint safety representatives. If they all did so situations would be created that would cause undue disruption of work and bring health and safety into disrepute. The guidance notes suggest that to avoid such problems agreement should be reached between trade unions so that the numbers of representatives are restricted to appropriate levels. A typical arrangement found in practice is for all the teachers at one LEA school to be represented by, say, an ATL appointee and for, say, an NAS/UWT member to represent all the teachers at another establishment. It is also common for a teacher safety representative to cover white collar staff where their union has not made an appointment. Blue collar unions sometimes prefer to appoint one safety representative to look after members at a number of schools run by a single employer. It must be emphasised that only trade unions can appoint safety representatives. Headteachers or governors cannot do so.

The functions of safety representatives

Arguably the most important function of a safety representative is to encourage cooperation between employers and employees in the promotion, development and monitoring of measures to ensure health and safety in the workplace. The regulations list a series of functions which a safety representative is expected to carry out:

(a) to investigate accidents, hazards and dangerous occurrences in the workplace (see "Accidents")
(b) to investigate complaints by constituents about matters relating to their health, safety and welfare at work
(c) to make representations to the employer about matters arising from such complaints and such investigations, and on general issues affecting health and safety in the workplace
(d) to carry out inspections of the workplace (see "Inspections")
(e) to represent constituents in consultations with enforcement authorities (see "HSE and enforcement in schools")
(f) to receive information that inspectors are required to provide
(g) to attend safety committees. (Safety representatives are not automatically *ex officio* members of a safety committee, membership being a matter for joint consultation: see "Safety Committees".)

Regulation 4(2) requires employers to allow safety representatives to take such time off with pay during working hours as is necessary to carry out the above listed functions and to undergo training.

Time off for safety representatives

The requirement to permit time off with pay for the carrying out of functions does not constitute a great problem in the non-teaching areas. An office worker or a caretaker can usually just leave work and it is waiting for them on their return. The position is different, however, where teaching staff are concerned, particularly in primary schools. It is not possible for a teacher to leave a class unsupervised for, say, 20 minutes and at a moment's notice. In practice safety representatives with a heavy teaching commitment usually find that the only time available to carry out such tasks is during their own breaks and lunchtime. This is scarcely time off with pay as specified in the legislation.

To address this problem one LEA negotiated a special facilities agreement with the teachers' associations. The basic concept was that the LEA allocated to each teacher safety representative a period of compensatory release from class contact each term in return for the time spent carrying out functions and also to permit an inspection to be carried out. The amount of time allocated depended on the size of the school. The associations were obliged to restrict the number of teachers appointed as safety representatives to a scale which, again, took account of the size of the school. The allocation was also subject to an inspection actually being carried out and a report being forwarded to the safety committee. The LEA undertook to provide a supply teacher to cover the release period, failing which a sum of money equivalent to the cost of a teacher for the period in question was credited to school funds. The agreed scale was as follows:

Size of school	Max. no. teacher safety representatives	Compensatory release days per term
Primary and nursery up to 350 pupils	1	1
Primary 350+ pupils	1	1.5
Secondary up to 999 pupils	1	2
Secondary 1000–1999 pupils	2	2 each
Secondary 2000+ pupils	3	2 each

Approved code of practice HSC 9 deals with time off for training. It says that safety representatives should be permitted time off with pay as soon as possible after appointment to attend a basic training course.

Basic training courses are run by the TUC (up to 10 days, one day per week), by individual unions (eg one teachers' association runs a five day residential course) and, occasionally, jointly by LEAs and the teachers' associations.

It is the responsibility of the trade union to provide relevant training. It must inform management of the course it intends to employ and provide on demand a copy of the syllabus. The union is also expected to give "at least a few weeks'" notice of the need to release an employee and must bear in mind factors such as the operational requirements of the employer.

Time off with pay for further training must be allowed where such training is necessary to meet "changes in circumstances or relevant legislation".

Regulation 11 provides for circumstances where an employer fails to grant a safety representative time off with pay for the purposes of receiving training, as per approved code of practice HSC 9, or to carry out the functions referred to above. Industrial tribunals are empowered to make a compensatory award which is "just and equitable in all the circumstances" and/or to order the employer to pay the safety representative any wages that have been withheld. Such cases must be brought before the industrial tribunal within three months of the failure occurring or within a reasonable period.

What is expected of a safety representative?

Safety representatives have the same legal responsibilities under HASAWA (s.7 and s.8) as any other employees but they cannot incur additional liability as a result of carrying out the specified functions. A safety representative may recommend or agree to a particular course of action but only management can actually decide what is to be done. Management have the authority, so they also have the responsibility.

Safety representatives are expected to take all reasonably practical steps to keep themselves informed about health and safety legislation, and in particular that relating to the work of their constituents. They should be aware of any particular hazards that might arise at their workplace and of the means necessary to eliminate or minimise them. They should be fully conversant with the employer's health and safety policy, organisation and arrangements. They are also expected to bring to the attention of management, either verbally or in writing, details of any conditions which are not safe or healthy, or of any unsatisfactory welfare provisions, that come to their notice.

Ultimately, they are responsible to their constituents and to the union that appointed them.

Information

Regulation 7 entitles safety representatives to inspect and take copies of any document relevant to the workplace and/or their constituents that the employer is required to keep by health and safety legislation (eg inspection reports relating to lifts) but not documents relating to the health of an identifiable individual. Employers are also required to make available to safety representatives information "within the employer's knowledge" that is "necessary to enable them to fulfil their functions". There are, however, a number of exclusions to this requirement, including:

(a) information obtained by the employer solely for purposes in connection with legal proceedings
(b) where disclosure of the information would cause substantial damage to the employer's undertaking
(c) where the information relates to an individual unless that person consents to disclosure.

Employers should provide safety representatives with information, such as:

(a) information kept about accidents, notifiable industrial diseases and dangerous occurrences, including any statistical records relating to these matters
(b) the results of any measurements taken to check the effectiveness of arrangements to protect health and safety (eg air test results after asbestos works)
(c) information provided under s.6 HASAWA by manufacturers and suppliers about articles and substances used at work
(d) technical information about hazards to health and safety, and the precautions necessary to avoid or minimise them, arising from the use of machinery, plant, equipment, etc
(e) information about any proposed changes that may affect the health

and safety at work of the employees (eg alterations, adaptations and extensions to the premises, the installation of new equipment).

Consultation, facilities and assistance

An amendment to these regulations was made by virtue of Regulation 17 of the Management of Health and Safety at Work Regulations 1992 (MHSWR). Regulation 4A now added to the Safety Representatives and Safety Committee Regulations 1977 spells out additional employers' duties towards safety representatives. Employers must consult with safety representatives "in good time" with regard to:

(a) the introduction of any measure which may substantially affect the health and safety of the safety representative's constituents
(b) the arrangements for the appointment of consultants or the nomination of in-house persons, to meet requirements of MHSWR
(c) any information required by health and safety legislation to be provided to the safety representative's constituents
(d) the planning and organisation of any training required by health and safety legislation to be provided to constituents
(e) the health and safety consequences for constituents of the planning for and introduction of new technologies into the workplace.

Regulation 4A(2) requires employers to provide "such facilities and assistance as safety representatives may reasonably require" to carry out their statutory functions.

In schools "facilities and assistance" that might reasonably be required may include use of a telephone, use of a photocopier, use of typing services, provision of a noticeboard in the staff room, provision of storage for relevant papers, etc and, perhaps in exceptional circumstances, accommodation for meetings of constituents. Headteachers can insist that such facilities are used by safety representatives only for tasks directly related to their role. Exactly what is provided will vary from school to school. For example, it would be reasonable to allow occasional use of typing services in a school where a typist is employed but it would not be reasonable to expect this otherwise.

Advice

Health and safety problems arise in schools from time to time that warrant the seeking of advice from external sources. LEAs may be able to provide the necessary expertise in areas such as structural engineering, environmental health, mechanical engineering and medicine. If an expert is to be asked to arbitrate on a matter of dispute, the school and the safety representative should agree who that expert is to be.

If safety representatives wish to call in their own technical advisor this must be agreed in advance by the employer. (The employer may wish to ensure that the proposed technical advisor is trained and qualified in the relevant discipline before giving such permission. Experience has shown that being an enthusiastic campaigner does not necessarily mean that an individual is technically competent.) A copy of any report made to the safety representative in such circumstances should be given to the employer.

Safety Committees

S.2(7) of HASAWA requires employers in "prescribed cases" to establish a safety committee if requested to do so by safety representatives. Regulation 9 specifies that this means when two safety representatives make such a request in writing. Within three months the employer must consult with those safety representatives and with representatives of the recognised trade unions having members at the workplace, post a notice stating the composition of the committee where it can be seen by all employees, and establish the committee.

Detailed advice on the various aspects of setting up and manning a safety committee are given in the guidance notes. Employers and safety representatives are advised to interpret the needs of the particular workplace and to develop a safety committee that takes full account of the relevant circumstances. Despite the title, a safety committee should cover all matters relating to health, safety and statutory welfare at the workplace. Whilst conceding that there may be a place for committees at "group or company" level the notes say that they will be most effective at grass roots level.

Objectives and functions

The main function of a safety committee is to keep under review the arrangements taken to secure health and safety in the workplace. The most important objective is the promotion of cooperation between the employer and employees in the instigation, development and implementation of measures aimed at achieving the health and safety at work of all employees. The notes recommend that committees should consider drawing up agreed objectives or terms of reference. They suggest that functions might include:

(a) considering reports and information provided by Health and Safety Executive (HSE) inspectors
(b) considering reports of workplace inspections and any other relevant reports that safety representatives may wish to submit
(c) studying accident statistics and trends so that recommendations can be made to management on corrective action
(d) assisting in the development of safety rules and safe systems of work
(e) monitoring the adequacy of the health and safety content of employee training
(f) monitoring communication and publicity relating to health and safety in the workplace
(g) providing a link with the enforcing authority.

The notes emphasise that responsibility for any necessary executive action to secure health and safety, and for the existence of adequate arrangements, remains with management. The work of a safety committee should supplement the efforts of management but can in no way be a substitute for them.

Membership

The membership and structure is a matter for consultation. The aim is for as compact a body as is compatible with adequate representation of the interests of management and the employees. Management representatives (the number of whom should not exceed the number of employees' representatives) are expected to have "adequate authority" and knowledge of the employers policies, etc.

Safety representatives are not automatically *ex officio* members, and they are not responsible for or to the committee.

Specialists who have relevant knowledge that would be of assistance from time to time may be co-opted for particular meetings.

Conduct of meetings

The guidance notes stress that the frequency of meetings should be determined by the volume of business, which will depend on the size of the workplace and the degree of risk inherent. Notices of the dates of meetings should be published where all employees can see them, and a copy of the agenda and any accompanying papers should be sent to all members at least a week before each meeting. Committees may wish to draw up rules for conduct of meetings and "it might be useful to appoint subcommittees to study particular health and safety problems".

Safety committees in schools

It is regrettable that some schools do not have safety committees. Where committees have been set up so that they operate in a way that is commensurate with the scale of the problems faced they have proved to be capable of making a very cost effective contribution to health and safety in schools. It is, however, important that matters are kept in proportion. In a small nursery school there may only be a need for the head, the teacher safety representative and the caretaker to meet for, say, 20 minutes each term to cover all necessary business. In a large secondary school a more formal approach is warranted, but it has to be remembered by everyone involved that safety committees are a means to a worthwhile end, not an end in themselves.

While the regulations require that a committee be established on request, as described above, this does not preclude headteachers from setting one up, and in some schools they are asked to do so by the governors. A report of the proceedings of school safety committee meetings are usually submitted to the subsequent meeting of the school governors.

The terms of reference for school safety committees should be a matter for consultation but the following example may be used as a framework for discussions.

Longmeads Junior School—Safety Committee

(a) The committee shall meet once per term. (Additional meetings will be held where circumstances warrant them, subject to agreement between the headteacher and the staff representatives.)

(b) The committee will consist of the headteacher, who will chair meetings, the caretaker (who will also represent the cleaning staff), the teacher safety representative and the head of kitchen. Other members of staff will be invited to attend meetings where appropriate. The school secretary will act as clerk.

(c) Colleagues from the Longmeads Adult Education Institute will be invited to attend meetings as necessary to discuss issues of mutual concern.

(d) The objective of this committee is to promote cooperation between all employees at the school with a view to achieving and maintaining a safe and healthy workplace for staff and pupils.

(e) The following will be standard agenda items:

(i) discussion of all accidents which have occurred since the last meeting, and of any remedial action that was taken to prevent a recurrence

(ii) the arrangement for the next termly inspection of the premises and consideration of any matters arising from the previous inspection

(iii) consideration of the implementation in the school of any new safety instructions advice issued by the LEA, DES, etc

(iv) consideration of progress on remedying any hazards which may have been identified

(v) to receive a report on fire drills held since the last meeting, and to discuss any matters arising

(vi) at each autumn term meeting, to review the content of the school's statement of health and safety arrangements, and to monitor its implementation.

(f) Meetings will not be minuted but action sheets will be prepared by the school secretary. They will be displayed on the school notice board and copies wll be made available to the next ordinary meeting of the school governors.

Further reading

Safety Representatives and Safety Committees, HSC, HMSO

Chapter 6
Accidents

One dictionary says that an accident is "an event without apparent cause, a chance mishap". If this is the case we are all in the hands of fate and any efforts to reduce accidents are bound to be unsuccessful. In reality, virtually no accident can be attributed exclusively to bad luck. There are certainly some accidents which are not preventable without restricting people's activities to an unacceptable degree, given the minor nature of likely consequences (eg pupils bumping into each other in the playground). There are also accidents whose causes are so unforeseeable that it would not be reasonable to take precautions against them. Nonetheless, most accidents are preventable, or their effects can be minimised, by reasonable precautions, but it is necessary to have some appreciation of the causes of accidents if appropriate measures are to be devised and applied.

There are various theories about accident causation. One of the simplest is particularly appropriate in schools, given the large population of persons who are inexperienced and physically immature. It suggests that people are likely to have an accident when placed in a situation with which they are not competent to cope. They may not be competent physically (eg not be strong enough, have reactions that are too slow, have defective eyesight) or from a skills aspect (ie lacking in training and/or experience). Other factors such as over-familiarity, fatigue, drugs and alchohol may also be relevant.

When an accident or a near miss occurs it is important to try to establish the precise cause because, otherwise, remedial measures taken to prevent a recurrence may be irrelevant. It will often be the case that there are several contributing causes of an accident. It will also be found that some of the accident producing behaviour is perpetrated not only by persons other than the injured party, but also by persons remote in distance and time from the scene (eg a pupil runs into a window which breaks, cutting his arm. Apart from local causes the lack of competence of the architect who specified such glass in such a position is clearly an important cause).

Studies in industry showed that there was a statistical relationship between the numbers of major injuries, minor injuries and near misses in the ratios of 1–29–300. These ratios vary according to the type of work involved, and even for different people, but the important points are that the vast majority of accidents do not cause major injury, but that if enough minor injuries and near misses occur, it is statistically likely that a major injury will happen. When a major injury does occur various external agencies are likely to descend upon the school to carry out investigations and make recommendations designed to prevent a similar accident happening again. In most cases, however, it is highly likely that investigation of minor injury and near miss accidents in the past would have produced similar recommendations long before the major injury occurred and may well have prevented it.

All accidents, whether or not they result in injury, should be reported to the headteacher. An investigation should be made to try to establish causes and careful consideration be given to remedial measures. (In specialist areas, such as science, CDT or Home Economics, it is sensible to delegate this task to the HoD.) Failure to adopt such an approach will mean that valuable and painfully gained experience is being ignored and, although some expenditure of time may be involved, it will be as nothing to the time that will be spent dealing with a major injury case.

One of the functions of a safety representative is to investigate dangerous occurrences and the causes of accidents at the workplace. Headteachers therefore need to ensure that safety representatives are informed of any incidents or accidents involving their constituents or the areas where their constituents work. While the intention of the legislation was not for investigations by safety representatives to be instead of those carried out by management, headteachers may consider in some instances that it would be more sensible for a single investigation on behalf of both management and staff to be made. Provided that the safety representative is agreeable to this, such an approach may well prove to have advantages.

Where major injuries are involved the Health and Safety Executive and/or the LEA safety advisor may wish to visit the site and carry out an investigation. It is therefore important to avoid disturbing the site until they have indicated that it is permissible to do so.

Accident Investigation

The following points should be borne in mind when carrying out an investigation:

(a) Avoid careless interviewing techniques when obtaining information from witnesses. (Do not ask questions that can be answered "yes" or "no". Do not ask questions in such a way that the witness is led into saying what the questioner appears to want to hear.)

(b) It is usually preferable for the witness to be allowed to tell the whole story without interruption, then to be guided back to those areas where clarification is needed.

(c) Establish whether witnesses actually saw what happened or if they saw the outcome of the accident and inferred subsequently what had led up to it.

(d) Remember that some witnesses may be unwilling to give accurate information because of fears of being blamed in some way, or of being disloyal to colleagues. (Explain that the reason for the investigation is to try to avoid a recurrence.)

(e) Do not jump to conclusions, no matter how obvious they may appear to be.

(f) Use an *aide-mémoire* to ensure that all relevant information is collected. All the points listed below will not be relevant in every case:

(i) Where did the accident happen?

(ii) When did the accident happen?

(iii) Who was injured?
Nature of injury.
Site of injury.

(iv) Who else was involved?

(v) Who witnessed the accident?

(vi) What was the injured person doing at the time of the accident? Was the person's action habitual/occasional/rare? If not usual, why was the person doing it?

(vii) Was the person working under pressure or to a deadline? Were there any relevant environmental factors?

(viii) Were protective measures available and appropriate? Were they used? If not, why not?

(ix) Was the person adequately trained to do the activity that resulted in injury?

(x)   Was there supervision in force? If not, should there have
        been? Was it adequate?
(xi)   Was a defect or design fault in the premises involved? If so,
        are similar situations to be found elsewhere in the building?

The amount of time and effort put into an investigation should be proportional to the potential severity of the consequences of any recurrence,
not to the severity of injury in the case itself.

Accident Recording and Reporting

The Reporting of Injuries, Diseases and Dangerous Occurrences Regulations 1985 established a system for the collection by the Health and
Safety Executive (HSE) of information about major injuries, occupational
diseases and certain workplace occurrences. In addition to providing the
HSE with statistical information to assist it in fulfilling its accident and
ill health prevention role, the system also provides an effective means of
ensuring early notification to it of those incidents which may warrant a
site visit by one of the inspectors.

The regulations require employers to report immediately the following
incidents:

(a) major injury or condition or death of an employee while at work,
    or death of an employee within a year as a result of a work incident
(b) major injury or condition or death of a visitor, pupil, etc while at
    a workplace or as a result of workplace activities
(c) an employee suffering one of the scheduled notifiable diseases
(d) injuries to an employee resulting in absence from work for three or
    more days after the day of the incident
(e) certain scheduled dangerous occurrences, whether or not injury is
    caused.

Incidents in categories (a) (b) and (e) must be reported to the HSE by
telephone, followed by submission of written details on Form F2508
within seven days.

"Major injuries or conditions" are:

(a) fracture of the skull, spine, pelvis, any bone in the arm or wrist (but not the hand) and any bone in the leg or ankle (but not the foot)

(b) amputation of a hand, foot, finger, thumb or toe, or part thereof if the joint or bone is severed

(c) the loss of the sight of an eye or a penetrating injury or a chemical or hot metal burn to the eye (minor irritations which are resolved with eye irrigation need not be reported)

(d) any injury requiring immediate medical treatment, or if consciousness is lost, as a result of an electric shock or electric burn

(e) loss of consciousness because of lack of oxygen

(f) any acute illness requiring immediate medical treatment, or if consciousness is lost, resulting from exposure to a substance

(g) acute illness requiring medical treatment where there is reason to believe that it resulted from exposure to a pathogen or infected material

(h) any other injury that results in the casualty being admitted immediately into hospital for more than 24 hours.

"Dangerous occurrences" include:

(a) the collapse or overturning of any scaffold

(b) the explosion, collapse or bursting of a vessel the contents of which are under pressure (eg steam boilers, gas cylinders, air receivers fed by a compressor) which results in significant damage to equipment or which might have injured someone

(c) an electrical short circuit or overload attended by fire or explosion which results in stoppage of the plant involved for more than 24 hours and which might have injured someone

(d) a fire or explosion which results in the stoppage of the plant involved or normal work in the area for more than 24 hours if it was due to the ignition of materials or their by-products (including waste) used in a work process or finished product

(e) the unintended collapse of any wall or floor in a workplace, or the collapse of any part of a building under construction

(f) any incident where plant or equipment comes into contact with an uninsulated overhead electric line at over 200 volts, or causes an electrical "flash" by coming close to it

(g) the collapse, overturning of or failure of a load-bearing part of a lifting device, such as a lift, hoist or crane

(h) the accidental release or escape of any substance or pathogen in circumstances which might cause death, major injury or condition or other damage to the health of any person.

Reportable diseases

The long schedule of reportable diseases accompanying the regulations include very few conditions that might arise from work in schools. These are:

(a) occupational asthma arising from work with animals or insects, or with epoxy resin materials
(b) leptospirosis arising from handling animals or work in areas infested by rats (eg ponds or waterways)
(c) hepatitis arising from work involving exposure to human blood products or body secretions and excretions.

There is no statutory requirement to report injuries to pupils or visitors which do not fall into the other "major injury or condition" categories but result in absence from "work" for three days, or if such persons contract a reportable disease at school. The Education Service Advisory Committee has, however, set up a voluntary scheme in the interests of collecting data of value to both the Health and Safety Executive and education employers. This scheme is described in a booklet published by HMSO in 1986 (see "Further reading").

The HSE does not require reports in respect of pupil injuries arising from collisions, slips and falls in playgrounds unless they are caused by the condition of the premises (eg pot holes, ice, worn steps), by plant or equipment being on the premises (eg contractors' machinery) or by a lack of proper supervision.

Activities away from school

Fatalities and major injuries to pupils occurring on school sponsored or controlled activities away from the school (eg field trips, holidays in the United Kingdom, sporting activities) must be reported if the accident arose out of, or in connection with, such activities.

In many LEAs the system is for schools to pass information about serious accidents, etc to central management who determine whether they are "reportable" and, where appropriate, pass on the details to the HSE. Where this is not the situation, and in establishments such as independent schools, it is essential that foolproof arrangements are maintained to ensure compliance with the requirements of these regulations. It is wise to adopt the approach that if any doubt exists about whether an incident should be reported, it should be reported. Failure to report incidents is a not uncommon cause of prosecutions.

Injuries on the premises

In addition to the statutory reporting requirements, records need to be kept of all injuries to pupils, staff and visitors that happen on the premises. Such records will be needed in the event of subsequent claims for compensation, for submission to each ordinary governors' meeting, and to assist in the management of the school. The latter reason is undoubtedly the most important but, sadly, although the information is usually available, it is rarely used for this purpose. Accident records over a period of two or three years give an accurate indication of where the main problem areas of a school lie and also allow decisions about expenditure on safety to be made on an informed basis. The effectiveness of any precautionary measures introduced can also be objectively assessed. Where finance has to be bid for from outside the school, statistically based justification will be found to be much more powerful than anecdotal evidence.

LEAs usually have an internal injury/accident reporting system, sometimes with a cut off that avoids details of the most minor injuries to pupils being forwarded to the authority. Where this is so schools can keep a copy of the system reports as part of their records and arrange for a simpler method to record the minor cases. All that would be required is:

(a) the name of the injured person
(b) the nature of the injury
(c) when, where and how it occurred
(d) who was supervising
(e) the treatment given.

There is yet another statutory requirement for accident record keeping. The Social Security Act 1985 requires that a book (Form BI 510, available from HMSO) is kept at each workplace and that details of injuries to employees are entered. Failure to comply may prevent an individual from subsequently obtaining industrial injury benefit.

Further reading

Reporting an Injury or Dangerous Occurrence, HSE 11 (rev.) 1986
Reporting a Case of Disease, HSE 17, 1989
Reporting School Accidents, HSE 1990
Guidance on a Voluntary Scheme for the Collection, Collation and Analysis of Injury, Disease and Dangerous Occurrence Data in the Education Sector, HMSO 1986
A Guide to the Reporting of Injuries, Diseases and Dangerous Occurrences Regulations 1985, HS(R) 23, HMSO 1986
Farmer D *Classic Accidents*, Croner 1990

Chapter 7

Inspections

Experience indicates that formal health and safety inspections are not often carried out in some schools, and that in others such exercises are not particularly effective. The problem appears to be that in the former cases the value of inspections has not been fully appreciated and in the latter they are not being carried out for the correct purposes.

With the exception of a few specialist areas in secondary establishments and kitchens, schools are not particularly hazardous places. Such hazards that do arise are significant because schools are intensively used by particularly vulnerable people. It can be shown statistically that a hazard will cause an accident once for every "x" number of times people are exposed to it. It is therefore essential that in schools hazards are identified quickly and dealt with. To achieve this all members of staff should be checking for hazards as they go about their work and any matters that they see and report should trigger an immediate response. (It is not possible, for example, for a broken window to be repaired immediately but the caretaker can quickly eliminate danger by boarding it up pending replacement.)

It can be seen that if, say, once a term an inspection is made with a view simply to collecting a list of hazards it will not be a very effective way of preventing accidents. There is also the risk, human nature being what it is, that staff noticing hazards in the weeks prior to the exercise may not take the trouble to report them in anticipation of the problem being picked up on the inspection.

Inspections will make a positive contribution to the safety of schools if any hazards found are recognised as symptoms of possible failures in the implementation of the school's arrangements or in the arrangements themselves. If, say, an area of defective carpet is found, questions should be asked to determine:

(a) how long it has been defective
(b) if it has been reported
(c) if not, the reason for this
(d) if it has, why has no short term remedial action (eg by the caretaker to minimise the tripping hazard) been taken?

(In 1991 a 10-year-old pupil suffered permanent head injuries when a school gate fell onto her head. The gate had been propped against a barrier for two months after being knocked off by a vehicle. The local authority was fined £1000 for failing to maintain safe premises. There had been a previous accident to a teacher involving the dismounted gate.)

Monitoring and Awareness

With this approach the inspection is effectively monitoring the carrying out of the school's arrangements and also raising the awareness of staff of the need to deal with hazards quickly. For headteachers, further benefits will accrue from their taking the opportunity to demonstrate to staff the importance that they place on health and safety matters. In secondary schools it is necessary for the task of inspecting specialist practical areas to be delegated to heads of department, but all other parts of the school should be inspected by a senior member of the school's management.

Safety representatives

Safety representatives are entitled to inspect workplaces used by their constituents provided that the headteacher has been given reasonable notice in writing of their intention to do so and they have not carried out an inspection within the prevous three months. More frequent inspections can be carried out by agreement with the headteacher if there has been a substantial change in working conditions (eg the provision of a temporary classroom), or if new information about hazards in schools has been published by the Health and Safety Commission (HSC) or the Health and Safety Executive (HSE). Headteachers are required to provide "such facilities and assistance as the safety representatives may reasonably require for the purpose of carrying out an inspection". This would include providing for private discussions with their constituents, but management can be present during the inspection if they so wish.

In practice, because schools work on a three term year, safety representatives usually carry out only three inspections per year. The HSC's guidance notes say that safety representatives should coordinate their work to avoid duplication and that the numbers of safety representatives carrying out an inspection is a matter for agreement between themselves and the headteacher. In larger schools where there is more than one safety representative it is common practice for the premises to be divided between them for inspection purposes.

Some trade unions, particularly those with few members at any one school, prefer to appoint a "peripatetic" safety representative to cover a number of establishments. This arrangement can cause problems where all the schools concerned do not have the same employer. With the special exceptions of those appointed by Equity and the Musicians' Union, safety representatives have no rights to inspect the premises of another employer. Where, for example, an LEA caretaker is appointed as a peripatetic safety representative covering a number of schools they must all be LEA, rather than voluntary aided, schools. There is, however, nothing to stop "other employers" agreeing to such situations should they so wish.

The HSC has said that it sees advantages in joint management/safety representative inspections being made. This approach has much to recommend it in schools, particularly in smaller establishments.

Research

A little time spent on research before an inspection is carried out will be amply repaid. Previous inspection reports should be read so that a check can be made to see that listed hazards have been remedied. If it has been decided that it would not be reasonably practicable to deal with a particular problem it is worthwhile to check whether there has been any change in circumstances that might warrant reconsideration of that decision. The hazard may have become worse or there may have been accidents or near misses. Accident reports should also be studied because they can accurately indicate possible problem areas that may be specific to that school.

The hazards that should be looked for are described in detail in the later chapters of this book. However, most accidents in schools are slips, trips and falls and the section on this subject is essential reading before each inspection.

Environmental factors

It should be borne in mind that environmental conditions can vary widely over the year and during the day. Staff working in each area should be asked about the adequacy of lighting at four o'clock on a winter's day, whether the heating is satisfactory, and if excessive temperatures are experienced on a summer's day. Enquiries should be made about extraneous noise problems, perhaps due to low flying aircraft or the school steel band practising next door.

External areas, and in particular access ways, should also be inspected. While pot holes and uneven paving slabs and drain covers are easily identified, other matters should be closely looked at, such as is the lighting adequate late on a January day, and what happened the last time that it snowed?

From time to time detailed check lists have been produced for people carrying out inspections of school premises. Comprehensive lists are very long and inclined to produce a blinkered approach. It is better, having carried out the above recommended research and read about the subject, to restrict oneself to a simple prompt list (eg housekeeping, floors, glass, lighting, heating, etc). When entering any room one should take a long, slow look around for anything that is unusual. Finally, it is necessary to question the people working in the area to see how they perceive their working conditions. Questions should be asked about anything that is seen but not understood.

Where safety inspections are concerned teacher safety representatives need be mindful of their professional code of conduct. They should consult with senior colleagues and, in particular, heads of department before making an inspection and should subsequently discuss their findings before deciding whether and in what terms to submit a written report to the headteacher.

Inspection forms

Specimens of suitable forms for use by safety representatives to record that an inspection has been made and to report to the headteacher details of any problems found on the inspection are included in the Guidance Notes on the Safety Representatives and Safety Committee Regulations 1977. Copies of these forms may be purchased from HSE offices.

The suggested form includes a column for completion by the head-teacher. Details of the remedial action taken, or brief reasons why it has been decided not to take any action, must be filled in, signed and a copy of the form returned to the safety representative within a reasonable period of time. Where the headteacher is unable to give a written response because the matter is one controlled by the LEA or the governors, a copy of the form should be forwarded by the headteacher to the representative of the employer who has the authority to complete and sign it. (It is not unknown for a headteacher having difficulties obtaining information or decisions from an LEA to ask a safety representative for a formal report about the matter so that a written response can be obtained!)

Where joint inspections are carried out, such formality may not be necessary. It is usual for a joint report about the findings of the inspection and any corrective action arising from it to be presented to the next meeting of the school safety committee, or where such does not exist, to the next staff meeting.

Further reading

The Regulations on Safety Representatives and Safety Committees, Approved Code of Practice and Guidance Notes, HSC

Chapter 8

Workplace (Health, Safety and Welfare) Regulations 1992

Since 1975 schools have been subject to the general requirements of s.2 of the Health and Safety at Work, etc Act but, unlike factories and offices, there has been no direct legislation spelling out what is meant by terms such as "adequate facilities for welfare at work". The practice of borrowing standards applying in factories and offices has proved less than ideal but better than nothing. These regulations signal an end to all such confusion.

Producing a single piece of legislation covering virtually every type of workplace must have been an unenviable task but the result is a standard for premises which can be readily applied in schools.

For most school premises most of the regulations will not apply until 1 January 1996. It is recommended that when the formal assessment required by the Management of Health and Safety at Work Regulations 1992 is carried out the "competent person" is asked also to prepare a detailed report of those changes which will be required to achieve compliance.

The following summary is likely to be adequate for most purposes but it is strongly recommended that a copy of *Workplace Health, Safety and Welfare*, which includes regulations, the Approved Code of Practice and guidance notes, is available in the health and safety library (see "Information") of every school.

Regulations 5–16 and 18–27 apply to new schools taken into use for the first time after 31 December 1992, and to any areas of existing schools subject to modification, extension or conversion where work commenced after that date. They apply to existing school premises from 1 January 1996. Regulation 17 applies to all schools from 1 January 1993.

Regulation 4 spells out the responsibility of employers and persons who control premises to ensure compliance with the regulations. (The requirements of other legislation such as The Management of Health and Safety at Work Regulations 1992 (MHSWR) to assess hazards and to consult safety representatives must be borne in mind when planning such compliance.)

Maintenance of Workplaces

Regulation 5 requires that the workplace, and any "equipment, devices and systems" provided there to comply with these regulations, must be kept clean, in an efficient state, in efficient working order and in good repair. Where it is appropriate a suitable system of maintenance must be established.

"Efficient" means from a health, safety and welfare viewpoint. "Equipment, devices and systems" requiring maintenance arrangements will include fencing, window cleaning access equipment or devices, escape lighting and ventilation systems (see "Engineering Inspections"). Arrangements should be made in advance to ensure that in the event of any defect occurring repairs are carried out properly and, where there is a technical breach of these regulations, eg a WC out of service, without delay. The advice of the person carrying out assessments under the MHSW Regulations should be sought on the detailed application of this regulation to specific premises.

Ventilation

In order to comply with Regulation 6 provision must be made to enable workplaces to be ventilated with fresh or purified air so that stale air, and/or air which is hot or humid because of a work process, is replaced at a reasonable rate.

In most areas of schools this requirement will be met by the provision of openable windows. In kitchens, home economics and CDT areas extraction of steam, excess heat and fumes, ideally from a point as close to the source as possible, may well be necessary. In totally enclosed buildings air conditioning systems must be maintained to a high standard to ensure that the circulated air is pure.

Temperatures, Lighting and Cleanliness

The temperature in indoor workplaces must be reasonable, and the method of heating such as to avoid the escape into the workplace of injurious or offensive fumes, gas or vapour. Thermometers must be available to staff to check the workplace temperature (Regulation 7).

The ACOP suggests that for sedentary work the minimum temperature that would be considered reasonable is 16°C. It warns of the need to ensure that combustion type heaters have an adequate air supply, and that paraffin and liquefied petroleum gas heaters do not produce harmful or offensive fumes. A reasonable level of provision of thermometers would be one for every four or five classrooms. ("Reasonable" temperatures in areas used by children will be higher, see "Temperatures".)

Workplaces must have suitable and sufficient lighting and such lighting will, so far as is reasonably practicable, be natural light. (Regulation 8, see "Lighting".)

Regulation 9 requires that workplaces, and all furniture, furnishings and fittings are kept "sufficiently clean". Walls, floors and ceilings must have surfaces which are capable of being kept clean. Waste materials must not be allowed to accumulate in the workplace.

Most areas of schools will be unacceptable from an aesthetic viewpoint long before lack of cleaning constitutes a risk to health and safety, though litter can cause slips and falls. The guidance notes suggest that floors should be cleaned once per week. Walls and ceilings "that can be reached with a 5 metre ladder" should be cleaned at suitable intervals. In areas where food is prepared, or in sanitary accommodation a good level of hygiene is required to minimise the spread of infection, and "sufficiently clean" will mean a much higher standard than in classrooms. Workplace surfaces must be specified with "cleanability" in mind. In workshops, for example, it may be necessary to seal floors to avoid permanent contamination with oil. (See "Cleaning in Pottery Areas".)

Working Space

Regulation 10 specifies that every room where employees work for other than short periods shall have sufficient height, floor area and unoccupied space for purposes of health, safety and welfare. Generally, this means that rooms must not be overcrowded. It should be possible readily to get to a work station and to get around the room with ease. The ACOP gives examples, but specifically excludes "rooms used for lectures, meetings and similar purposes", while pupils are not covered by this regulation. If the volume of an empty workroom (disregarding any height above 3 m) is divided by the number of employees normally working there the minimum acceptable result is 11 m^3. If the room contains much furniture this minimum may be insufficient.

Workstations

Regulation 11 spells out that every workstation must be suitable for any employee (including any with disabilities) in the workplace who is likely to work there, and for any work that might be carried out there. It specifies the need for ready access and egress and the need to avoid slipping and tripping hazards in the vicinity. It also requires provision of suitable seating where the work can or must be done in a sitting position. Seating must be suitable for the person using it and for the work to be performed, and a footrest must be provided for persons who cannot comfortably place their feet on the floor. In schools this regulation will have most relevance to persons such as headteachers, librarians and office workers. It is intended to ensure that desks and chairs are ergonomically designed to suit both users and the tasks that they undertake.

Where such workstations are used for word processing and microfiche reading, the Health and Safety (Display Screen Equipment) Regulations 1992 (HS (DSE) Regulations) may apply. If they do apply they will take precedence over these regulations. If those do not there is unlikely to be much difference in the workstation furniture needed by a typist working for, say, five hours per day and that prescribed in the HS (DSE) Regulations for an intensively working wordprocessor operator. Again, the advice of the competent person carrying out assessments under the MHSWR 1992 should be sought (see "Display Screen Equipment").

Floors

All floors and traffic routes in a workplace must be constructed so as to be suitable for their intended purpose. They shall have "no hole or slope, or be uneven or slippery so as, in each case, to expose any person to a risk to his/her health and safety". (Where adequate means have been taken to prevent falls "holes" may be disregarded, and account taken of any handrail provided when assessing whether such a risk exists because of a slope.) Suitable and sufficient handrails must be provided on staircases (Regulation 12). Where necessary floors must have an effective means of drainage. They must, so far as is reasonably practicable, be kept free of obstructions and from any article or substance that may cause someone to slip, trip or fall.

The ACOP says that where tripping hazards arise because of wear and tear adequate precautions should be taken until repairs are carried out. Moderate and steep slopes, and ramps for use by persons with disabilities, should be provided with a handrail as necessary. Floor surfaces likely to get wet should have a reasonable degree of slip resistance in that condition. "A slip resistant coating should be applied where necessary." It is important to ensure that flooring around machines is slip resistant, and to deal immediately with spillages of liquids (see "Slips, Trips and Falls", and "School Kitchens").

Falls from Heights

Regulation 13 specifies that, so far as is reasonably practicable, "suitable and effective" measures, are to be taken to prevent persons falling from heights or being struck by falling objects, where either event is likely to cause personal injury. Where it is reasonably practicable the measures taken must be other than personal protective equipment or training.

Secure fencing should be provided, (wherever it is possible to do so), at any place where a person might fall 2 m or more, or lesser heights where factors such as the possibility of falling onto sharp objects, or into the path of traffic, are present. Additional safeguards may be necessary if unauthorised access by pupils, etc is foreseeable. Detailed requirements in respect of fixed ladders, roof work and stacking and racking of objects and materials are specified in the ACOP.

Glazing

Any windows or panels of "translucent" material in doors or gates, which represent a hazard to health and safety, must be of safety material or be protected against breakage. Where there is a risk of persons colliding with glass panels because they are not immediately apparent, the panels must be marked to counter the risk (Regulation 14).

The ACOP says that all glass panels in doors, gates and side panels which are wider than 250 mm, and where any part of the panel is at shoulder level or below, should be of "safety material", or be protected by a barrier or screen to prevent contact with the glass. Windows, where any part of the glazed panel is below waist level, must also be of "safety material" or be similarly protected. "Safety materials" are defined in the ACOP as materials such as polycarbonate sheet, laminated and toughened glass, and annealed glass in panel sizes considered appropriate for its thickness. While these precautions would no doubt be sufficient in buildings used by adults, grim experience indicates that they are totally inadequate in schools. It is strongly recommended that any glazing below head height with which it is foreseeable that pupils may collide should, in the case of windows, be of "safety material" (and this should not be annealed glass), or be protected by the application of film in the case of annealed Georgian wired glass in doors specified for fire resistance purposes.

When it is necessary to mark large panels of glazing because they are not immediately apparent the marking must be conspicuous and be at a conspicuous height. Where a barrier is used to prevent someone going through glass and subsequently falling from a height the barrier must be constructed so that it is difficult to climb. The ACOP specifically excludes glasshouses from the above requirements (see "Glass Accidents").

Windows

Regulation 15 requires that it should be possible for someone to reach and operate the controls of windows, skylights and ventilators without risk to their health and safety. No window shall be in a position when open which puts at risk anyone's health and safety.

The current situation in some schools, where it is necessary to climb on furniture to operate windows, will need to be changed. Window controls should be located to minimise the possibility of a person falling through or out of the window. Where there is a possibility of someone falling out of a window on upper floors devices should be fitted to limit opening to a safe extent. (The bottom edge of opening windows should be at least 800 mm above floor level unless a barrier is fitted to prevent falls.) Where windows open into a playground so that there is a risk of collision some form of barrier will be needed to prevent accidents.

All windows and skylights shall be of a design or be so constructed that they may be cleaned safely. When assessing whether this requirement is met account can be taken of any special provisions which may have been made to facilitate safe cleaning (Regulation 16). (Special provisions include suspended cradles, anchorage points for safety harnesses, and tying or fixing points for ladders over 6 m long—maximum permitted ladder length is 9 m.)

Organisation of Traffic Routes

Regulation 17 is concerned with the organisation of foot and vehicular traffic routes in workplaces. Such routes must be suitable for the vehicles and persons (including persons with disabilities) who will use them. To be "suitable" there must be sufficient separation between foot and vehicular traffic where a route is shared, there must be sufficient separation between a vehicle route and doors, gates and foot traffic leading onto it, and both types of route must be usable without causing danger to the health and safety of persons at work nearby. All traffic routes shall be suitably indicated where it is necessary for reasons of health and safety. These requirements apply from 1 January 1993.

In schools the main areas requiring attention will be the interface between people and vehicles, and controlling the speed and routes of vehicles on the premises. Much will depend on the layout of the school grounds. In an ideal situation vehicles will use entry gates and roadways dedicated to their exclusive use, with ready access to car parks, delivery points and rubbish collection areas which are remote from areas used by pupils. In practice this will rarely be the case. A careful assessment of current arrangements should be made to identify all possible hazards arising from vehicle movements on the premises. Speed restrictions will significantly reduce otherwise unavoidable risks, and speed humps are an effective means of countering any disregarding of such limits. Where it is possible to do so vehicle routing should be planned to avoid the need for heavy vehicles to reverse, or to pass within 2 m of any building. In difficult situations it may be necessary to ban vehicles from moving on the site when pupils are arriving or departing; where regular deliveries/ collections are made schools may need to liaise with the organisations concerned so that vehicle movements are avoided at the beginning and end of the school day and during breaks.

Adequate supervision of pupils will be required to maintain any system devised for their protection.

Drivers of vehicles must be warned of possible hazards such as sharp bends, junctions, road humps, etc, and of speed restrictions by the use of signs complying with the Traffic Signs Regulations and General Directions 1981 and with the Highway Code. Where necessary road markings should also be used. On some school sites the provision of direction notices will allow drivers to go directly to their destination rather than wandering about. Sources of advice on these matters will include road safety officers employed by local authorities and the local police, although this may not strictly be within their remit.

Doors

In Regulation 18 the main point of interest to schools is that doors which swing in both directions, and conventionally hinged doors on main traffic routes, are required to be fitted with a viewing panel. The panel should be located such that a person in a wheelchair can be seen from the other side of the door. (The advice of the local fire authority should be sought before the fire resistance of doors is compromised by modifications.)

Regulation 19 is not relevant to schools.

Sanitary Accommodation

Regulations 20 and 21 deal with the provision of sanitary conveniences and washing facilities for employees at a workplace. Sufficient facilities must be provided at readily accessible locations. Washing facilities must be provided in the immediate vicinity of every sanitary convenience, even if minimum levels of such provision are already met elsewhere. Rooms containing these facilities must be adequately ventilated and lit, and be kept in a clean and orderly condition. Supplies of clean hot and cold, or warm, water must be available, and this must be running water unless that is technically impossible. Soap (or a suitable substitute) and towels (or other means of hand drying) must be provided. Separate facilities must be provided for men and women except where a convenience and wash basin are in a room with a door that can be locked from the inside and which is intended to be used by only one person at a time. However, washing facilities can be shared by men and women if they are provided for the washing of hands and face only.

The ACOP specifies the minimum level of provision considered "sufficient" but says that more facilities may be necessary if employees are limited to using them at set break times. If the level of provision does not permit access "without undue delay" it is insufficient. The following table shows the stated minimum levels. Where certain facilities are restricted in use to, say, men, women, headteacher, school-keeping staff or office staff a separate calculation should be made for each category of user.

Maximum number of employees on site at one time	Minimum number of water closets	Minimum number of washstations
1–5	1	1
6–25	2	2
26–50	3	3
51–70	4	4
76–100	5	5

Where employees' facilities are also used by members of the public provision should be increased as necessary to ensure access by employees "without undue delay".

Where sanitary accommodation is used only by men a proportion of the provision may be in the form of urinals, if it is so desired, on the following scale.

No. of men	No. of water closets	No. of urinals
1–15	1	1
16–30	2	1
31–45	2	2
46–60	3	2
61–75	3	3
76–90	4	3

Adequate privacy must be ensured for users. Each water closet must be enclosed and have a door that can be locked from within. It must not be possible for persons outside the facilities area to see urinals or showers when the entrance door is opened. If windows to these facilities are overlooked they must be fitted with frosted glass, blinds or curtains.

Where any employee has a disability any special provisions necessary to permit access and use of the facilities must be made.

Where work is particularly strenuous showers or baths should be provided. In schools this requirement will apply to staff engaged in physical education. (DES regulations require that sanitary accommodation and washrooms for staff use must be separate from that provided for pupils. For details of minimum provisions for pupils see The Education (School Premises) Regulations 1981.)

Drinking Water

An adequate supply of wholesome drinking water must be readily available for employees at work. It must be marked as drinking water by an appropriate sign where there is any possibility of confusion with other, "non-drinking", water supplies. A sufficient number of suitable cups, or similar drinking vessels, must be provided unless the supply is in the form of a drinking fountain (Regulation 22).

Drinking water should be obtained directly from the public mains supply. Where this is not technically possible a cistern supply is permissible provided that the cistern is properly covered, is regularly checked for cleanliness and is disinfected as necessary. So far as is reasonably practicable, drinking water taps should not be in water closets. Where non-disposable cups are provided means of washing them should be available nearby.

Work and Street Clothing

Regulations 23 and 24 describe the arrangements which must be made in respect of the street and work clothes of employees. Adequate accommodation must be provided for street clothes, and for special clothing that is worn at work but not taken home. Where it is reasonably practicable to do so facilities must be made available to dry street clothes and work clothing which has become wet. Changing facilities must be provided where employees have to wear special work clothing and have to remove more than their street clothes in order to change before starting work. Where changing rooms are necessary they must either provide separate facilities, or separate use of facilities, for men and women where necessary for reasons of propriety, and suitable security must be provided for the employees' own clothing.

"Special" clothing includes overalls, hats worn in kitchens, laboratory coats and track suits worn by physical education teachers. For most staff in schools the minimum requirement will be met with provision of an individual peg or hook on which to hang street clothes, located in a clean, dry, well ventilated place. Where work clothing becomes wet, and it is not possible to dry it before the start of the following day, fresh dry clothing will have to be provided. Where changing facilities are necessary provision of a lockable locker will meet the requirements for security. Changing facilities must be of adequate size to avoid overcrowding, be provided with sufficient seating and be adjacent to clothing accommodation and, where provided under Regulation 21, showers or baths.

Rest and Eating Facilities

Regulation 25 specifies the provision of separate rest rooms and eating facilities for workers whose workplace is too hazardous to allow rest breaks or meals to be taken there. It also requires that pregnant women and nursing mothers at work are provided with suitabile facilities for resting. Suitable and sufficient arrangements must also be made for employees who regularly eat meals in their workplace.

Whilst the requirement for rest rooms will not apply to schools, science and CDT teachers and technicians, and pottery and art teachers need to be allocated somewhere away from their work rooms to eat meals. If the school has a canteen and these members of staff can use it without any obligation to buy food compliance would be achieved. Employees who regularly eat meals in their workplaces must be provided with the means to prepare or obtain hot drinks (eg an electric kettle, a vending machine or a canteen). If hot food cannot be obtained in, or reasonably near to, the workplace some means of heating the employees' own food must also be provided. Where pregnant women and nursing mothers are at work they must be provided with somewhere to rest and lie down reasonably close to sanitary facilities. Although staff rooms are not covered by this regulation their provision is made a statutory requirement by DES Regulations (see "The Education (School Premises) Regulations").

Further reading

Workplace health, safety and welfare (Regulations, ACOP and Guidance Notes), HSE 1992, HMSO
Seating at Work, HS(G)57, HMSO 1991

Chapter 9

Provision and Use of Work Equipment Regulations 1992

The Provision and Use of Work Equipment Regulations 1992 (PUWER), represent a major change in health and safety legislation and will mean that for the first time the provision and use of much equipment in schools will be subject to specific legal requirements. In practice, however, those schools which have previously borrowed and applied appropriate industrial standards will have little difficulty in achieving compliance.

In the past legislation was introduced to deal with work equipment safety in individual industries, or in respect of particular types of machine. The new regulations draw together all those requirements, combine them with current good practice and apply the result to all workplaces, including schools. At the end of the transitional period which applies to some of the regulations (on 1 January 1997) 20 pieces of existing legislation will be wholly or partially repealed. The following description of the regulations and how they will apply to schools is necessarily brief. The Health and Safety Executive (HSE) publication *Work Equipment—Guidance on Regulations* provides 64 pages of detailed guidance with many illustrations and examples, and must be considered essential reading for heads of practical departments. A copy should also be available in the school health and safety library (see "Information").

"Work equipment" so far as these regulations are concerned means items such as lawn-mowers, computers, overhead projectors, guillotines, circular saws, ladders, photocopiers, laboratory apparatus, hammers, hand-saws, cook's knives, drill bits and fume cupboards. It also means such equipment provided by employees for use at work. Substances, parts of buildings (eg stairs) and private cars are not work equipment.

The regulations came into effect on 1 January 1993, except that equipment in schools on that date will not be subject to Regulations 11–24 until 1 January 1997. (The legislation "borrowed" by schools, such as the guarding requirements of the Factories Act, will remain in force until 1997 but it makes more sense for the similar standards described in Regulations 11–24 to be "borrowed" during the transitional period. If second-hand equipment is purchased from another employer the buyer will have to ascertain that it complies with Regulations 11–24, but equipment moved between two schools of an LEA would be considered to be existing equipment.)

The requirements of these regulations are imposed on employers in respect of their employees, on self-employed persons in respect of themselves, and on persons who control premises in respect of people who use work equipment there—but only to the extent of the person's control (Regulation 4). (In schools the latter requirement will apply to governors.)

Work Equipment

Work equipment must be suitable for the purpose for which it is used or provided. It must be selected with due regard to the working conditions and to the risks to the health and safety of persons which exist in the place where it will be used, and to any additional risks introduced by the use of the equipment. Employers must also ensure that equipment is only used for operations and in conditions for which it is suitable (Regulation 5).

In practice this means that the equipment will have been designed and produced for the work in question, and will be used in accordance with the manufacturer's instructions. The suitability from a health and safety viewpoint of the location or places of use of the equipment must be considered. Access to the place in question by pupils may be a problem, as may insufficient space safely to manipulate large dimensioned materials. When fitted with an appropriate blade a circular saw is suitable for ripping or cross cutting, but it is not suitable for rebating work.

Maintenance

Regulation 6 requires that work equipment is maintained so as to secure the health and safety of users. Where machinery has a maintenance log it must be kept up to date.

Apart from the obvious requirement to maintain guards, fences, covers, etc in good condition, the use of a blunt or chipped blade in a circular saw, or a "mushroomed" cold chisel, would be breaches of this regulation.

Specific Risk

Where work equipment involves a specific risk employers must ensure that its use is restricted to designated persons who have received adequate training (Regulation 7). In schools examples will be swimming pool dosing equipment (see "Swimming Pools") and woodworking machines (see "Woodworking Machines").

Information and Instructions

Employers are required by Regulation 8 to ensure that persons using work equipment and their supervisors and managers have available to them adequate and comprehensible information (and, where appropriate, written instructions) about the use of the equipment. Such information/instructions should include details of the conditions in which and the methods by which the equipment may be used, of foreseeable abnormal situations and the user's response should such arise, and any conclusions drawn from experience gained in the equipment's use. It must be remembered that this requirement is qualified by reasonable practicability. It is not necessary to give the caretaker information on how to use a screwdriver or a hammer: the risk would not justify the effort. Where there is a significant risk involved in the use of work equipment an employer will have to judge the extent of information that is needed, giving regard to the user's experience and training, to allow safe usage. Under s.6 Health and Safety at Work, etc Act manufacturers and suppliers are required to provide sufficient information to allow the correct installation, and the safe use and maintenance of equipment for use at work. The intention of this regulation is to ensure that such information is made available to users and their supervisors. Schools should try to obtain from manufacturers instruction sheets and manuals for existing equipment. These, and all future additions, should be kept in the school's health and safety library (see "Information"), and users briefed about their availability.

Training

Employers must ensure that persons using work equipment and their supervisors receive adequate training to secure health and safety, including proper methods of use, details of risks that may arise and of necessary precautions (Regulation 9).

In considering what is adequate, account must be taken of the difference between the employee's current level of competence and that required for safe use of equipment. Supervisors will not necessarily require training to the same standard as an operator: they must, however, have sufficient knowledge to be able to provide adequate supervision. In schools it is often the case that a technician is a qualified woodworking machinist but the HOD has only a vague knowledge of such work. The special training requirements in the Woodworking Machines Regulations 1974 and the Abrasive Wheels Regulations 1970, together with specific training requirements for young persons under various legislation (see "Work Experience"), will not be repealed in 1997.

Conformity with European Standards

Employees must ensure that any item of work equipment provided for use in the workplace after 31 December 1992 complies with British legislation implementing any relevant EC directive (Regulation 10(i)). This means that schools should specify "complying with British legislation implementing any relevant EC directive" when purchasing work equipment. Eventually all work equipment will be subject to a product directive, carry a "CE" mark and be sold, on request, with a copy of the EC Declaration of Conformity. If the work equipment complies with British legislation implementing a product directive then any corresponding requirements in Regulations 11–24 will not apply (Regulation 10(2)). (Once the product directives are fully in force—1 January 1995, so far as the Machinery Directive is concerned—only products conforming and carrying a "CE" mark may be marketed in the UK.)

Guarding of Machines

Regulation 11 requires employers to ensure that effective measures are taken to prevent access to any dangerous part of machinery or to any rotating stock bar, or to stop the movement of such parts before any person can be harmed by them. Prevention of access will be achieved by using fixed guards to enclose the dangerous parts or rotating stock bar where and to the extent that it is technically possible to do so. Where fixed guards are not technically possible adjustable guards or other protective devices will be provided to the extent that is technically possible, but where such measures are not completely effective jigs, holders, push sticks, etc will be provided. Where such provision is not totally effective operators must be given adequate information, instruction, training and supervision to secure their safety. All guards and devices must be suitable for their purpose, be of good construction, sound material and adequate strength, and be properly maintained. They must not cause increased risks, be easily bypassed or disabled, unduly restrict vision of the operation where such is necessary, and allow for safe maintenance and/or adjustment.

"Stock bar" means material projecting outside the lathe head-stock. "Dangerous part" is a part which presents a reasonably foreseeable risk of injury. These requirements are largely self-explanatory. In schools, circular saws provide a good example of the selection of preferred options. Below the table fixed guards are possible, and must be provided, but above the table such are not practicable. An adjustable crown guard is therefore fitted but this is not totally effective. Push sticks and holders must be provided but, as they do not give complete protection, adequate training, supervision, etc is also required.

Specified Hazards

Regulation 12 is concerned with certain specified hazards that may arise when work equipment is used. The hazards listed are:

(a) articles or substances falling or being ejected
(b) the rupture or disintegration of work equipment
(c) equipment overheating or catching fire
(d) the unintended or premature discharge of articles, gas, dust, liquid, vapour or substance which is produced, used or stored in the work equipment
(e) an unintended or premature explosion of the work equipment or a substance or article produced in it.

Employers must take measures to ensure that risks to the health and safety of persons arising from these hazards are eliminated, where it is reasonably practicable to do so, or else be adequately controlled. Measures such as the provision of personal protective equipment and training and supervision will only suffice if other precautions are not reasonably practicable. Where it is appropriate, measures to minimise the effects of the hazard, as well as steps to reduce the likelihood of occurrence, will be introduced. (Examples of such hazards in schools include abrasive wheels (b), fume cupboards (d), acetylene gas bottles (c), segmented work pieces in wood lathes (a), laboratory equipment (e).)

Unavoidable discharges or ejection, such as sawdust from a circular saw, are not covered by this regulation.

Heat and cold

Where work equipment, or articles or substances used or stored in it, are at high or very low temperatures, protection must be provided, where appropriate, in order to prevent burns, scalds or searing (Regulation 13).

In schools it would not be appropriate to provide protection for equipment such as irons, cooker hobs or soldering irons but, where the risk of injury is significant (for example in foundry work), protection will be required.

Controls and Control Systems

Regulations 14–18 cover the provision of controls and control systems for work equipment. They will mainly apply to powered work equipment with moving parts where controls are required for health and safety reasons. Some non-powered items may also require control facilities (eg brakes on trolleys or wheelchairs), as will some powered equipment without moving parts (eg kilns, ovens).

Work equipment must be provided with controls requiring deliberate operation to start and restart, and to change speed, temperature, pressure and/or power where such may have health and safety implications (Regulation 14). (Restarting of equipment should not be possible by just closing an interlocked panel, which means the provision of no-volt release devices.)

Work equipment must also be provided, where appropriate, with readily accessible controls to bring it to a complete stop and/or, where necessary for reasons of health and safety, switch off sources of energy after stopping the functioning of the equipment. Such controls must operate with priority over any other controls (Regulation 15). (The complete stop does not have to be instantaneous.)

Regulation 16 requires the provision of emergency stop controls where they are appropriate for health and safety reasons. Such controls are to have priority over controls provided in response to Regulation 15. (In school workshops such controls should be connected to control all machines in the areas simultaneously rather than individual machines.)

All controls for work equipment must be clearly visible and identifiable, with appropriate labelling where necessary. Unless it is unavoidable, controls must be positioned such as to avoid risk of injury when they are operated (Regulation 17(1) and (2)). Regulation 17(3) is concerned with ensuring that in circumstances where operation of a control could place other persons at risk the control is located to enable the operator to see the hazard, failing which a safe system of work or audible warnings must be provided. A good example in schools is the need for area gas cocks in laboratories, workshops etc to be labelled, and located in a sensible position. The requirements of 17(3) may also apply when lifts are being serviced, and may require delivery vehicles with poor rearward visibility to sound audible alarms when reversing.

Control systems for work equipment must, so far as reasonably practicable, be safe, and their operation (and any fault in, damage to or loss of power to the control system) must not result in an increased risk to health and safety. The control system must not impede the operation of stop or emergency stop controls (Regulation 18). This means that controls should be "fail safe" in design, with lo-volt release facilities built in if an unexpected restart would create danger, where such is reasonably practicable. Any interlocks fitted to a machine are part of the control system and, unlike many found on equipment such as woodworking lathes, should be of fail-safe design.

Isolation of Energy Sources

Regulation 19 requires the provision of suitable, clearly identifiable and readily accessible means, where appropriate, to isolate work equipment from its energy sources. Appropriate measures must be taken to avoid exposing work equipment users to danger when the energy source is reconnected. (Lo-volt release facilities will satisfy this last requirement in the case of machinery. When turning on a local gas supply cock to a laboratory area a physical check of all gas points will be required.)

Stability

Employers are required to ensure that work equipment, or any part of it, is stabilised by clamping or other means where necessary for health and safety reasons (Regulation 20).

Transportable, as opposed to portable, woodworking machines must be fastened down. Ladders should be tied or footed (see "Ladders and Steps") when in use. Access platforms used for stage lighting work must be stabilised by limiting height according to base dimensions or by fitting outriggers.

Lighting

Employers must ensure that suitable and sufficient lighting, which takes account of the operations being carried out, is provided where a person uses work equipment (Regulation 21).

General lighting will be adequate for many tasks but where necessary local lighting on the machine should be provided (eg lathes, sewing machines). Temporary lighting can be used in areas only occasionally used by maintenance staff (see "Lighting" and the Workplace (Health, Safety and Welfare) Regulations 1992).

Maintenance

Work equipment must be constructed or adapted in such a way that, so far as is reasonably practicable, maintenance can be carried out without risks to health and safety (Regulation 22).

There is unlikely to be any requirement for carrying out maintenance operations on work equipment in schools while the item is in use. Maintenance of electrical equipment is covered by the Electricity at Work Regulations 1989 (see "Electrical Safety").

Markings and Warnings

Regulation 23 requires that work equipment is marked in a clearly visible manner with any marking necessary for reasons of health and safety. Regulation 24 requires that work equipment incorporates unambiguous, easily seen and understood warnings or warning devices which are appropriate for reasons of health and safety.

In schools examples of markings will include the maximum rotation speed of abrasive wheels, the maximum safe working load on a lifting beam, the colour coding of gas cylinders, and signs on highly flammable liquid stores (see "Storage of Hazardous Materials"). Warnings and warning devices include prohibitions ("Machine only to be operated by John Green and Mary Brown"), signal lamps indicating "power on" or, perhaps, a fume cupboard fan failure, or an audible reversing alarm on a delivery vehicle.

Application in Schools

Schools with well chosen, well maintained work equipment should have little difficulty in complying with the requirements of these regulations. Existing equipment (that provided for use before 31 December 1992) is exempt from the requirements of Regulations 11–24 until 1 January 1997 but is likely to comply anyway unless it is old or of dubious manufacture.

The "competent person" carrying out the general assessment required by Regulation 3(1) of the Management of Health and Safety at Work Regulations 1992 should report on whether PUWER Regulations 5–9 are being complied with. It is recommended that the competent person also be asked to report on any failures to meet the requirements of PUWER Regulations 11–24 so that even if it is decided that immediate action is not required time is in hand to replace or modify the equipment before those regulations come into effect.

Schools purchasing new equipment should ensure that it complies with the required standard (see Regulation 10 above). Schools purchasing second-hand equipment after 1 January 1993 will have to ensure that it complies fully with Regulations 11 to 24 immediately. Hired or leased equipment obtained after 1 January 1993 is "second-hand" but the responsibility for checking compliance with Regulations 11–24 rests with the company owning the items.

Further reading

Work Equipment: Guidance on Regulations, HSE 1992, HMSO

Chapter 10
Safety

Slips, Trips and Falls

Analysis of accident statistics show that approximately a third of all staff injuries in schools result from slips, trips and falls. Even more significant is that about 80 per cent of all serious injuries to staff are caused in this way. From an accident prevention viewpoint floors are clearly an area worthy of attention.

A study of accident reports shows that the most frequent causes of slips, trips and falls are:

(a) Wet floors following cleaning. (Floor washing should be carefully planned so that a minimum number of people will need to use the area before the floor is dry. Warning signs should be put up at the limits of the wet area. Cleaners should work towards the doorway so as to avoid walking across wet areas.)

(b) Wet floors in entrances to the building during inclement weather. (Special absorbent mats, designed to stay flat and with bevelled rubber edges, will largely solve this problem, and keep the floors in the school cleaner as a bonus.)

(c) Wet floors due to spillage from kettles. (Where drinking water is not available in the areas where tea, etc is made, plastic stoppered containers should be used to fetch water.)

(d) Loose or torn carpets. (The caretaker should keep a reel of wide adhesive carpet tape to effect temporary repairs.)

(e) Moss, leaves and lichen on external paths.

(f) "Hidden" steps. (Where steps are close to doorways, blend into flooring so that they are not readily apparent, or are in badly lit areas, warning notices and or the use of a contrasting coloured paint on the tread edges should be considered. Teaching platforms may present similar problems.)

(g) Loose or missing floor tiles or paving slabs. (It is sometimes possible to rearrange furniture as a temporary expedient.)

(h) Oil or grease spills, particularly in kitchens, workshops and car parking areas.

(i) Use of inappropriate floor treatments. (The manufacturers of polishes, etc will usually give advice on the suitability of their product for a given type of surface.)

(j) Inadequate lighting. (This should be assessed in worst possible conditions, ie at four o'clock on a wet winter's day. Areas outside the building should not be forgotten.)

(k) Litter.

(l) Makeshift methods of reaching heights and inexpert use of ladders and steps (see "Ladders").

(m) Unsuitable footwear.

(n) Telephone and electrical cables laying across walkways. (Often caused by persons moving desks and tables without consideration of this problem. Wide adhesive tape will provide a temporary solution pending relocation of telephone points and mains sockets.)

(o) Objects left in walkways and corridors.

(p) Hurrying and inattention. (The traditional rule of "no running in corridors" makes a major contribution to accident prevention in schools.)

(q) Desk and filing cabinet drawers left open.

(r) Obscured vision when carrying bulky items.

(s) Badly fitting mats in mat wells in entrances. ("Dirt control" mats are much less likely to cause tripping hazards and will also reduce cleaning requirements.)

(t) Ice and snow. (Access paths must be kept safe by clearing and the use of salt).

Further reading

Watch Your Step: Prevention of Slipping, Tripping and Falling Accidents at Work, HSE, HMSO

Personal Protective Equipment at Work Regulations 1992

These regulations cover the provision of clothing and equipment intended to be worn or used by employees to protect their health and safety. They do not apply to ordinary working clothes, uniforms, competitive sports equipment, personal sirens/alarms, overalls and caps provided for food hygiene purposes, or to equipment provided in compliance with other current legislation such as the Control of Substances Hazardous to Health Regulations 1988 and the Noise at Work Regulations 1989.

Employers are required to provide personal protective equipment to employees exposed to risks to their health and safety unless those risks have been adequately controlled by other means. Such equipment must be appropriate for the risks involved, take account of any special requirements of the users (such as their state of health), fit the individual correctly, so far as is technically possible be capable of preventing or controlling the risk in question without increasing risk in general, and must comply with any appropriate, relevant legal standard for its design or manufacture.

Where the risk is such as to warrant the provision of personal protective equipment, no charge may be made on the employee.

Employers must ensure that personal protective equipment is maintained (including replacement and cleaning as necessary) in an efficient state, that appropriate storage is provided for it when it is not in use, and that employees are given adequate information, instruction and training about its use. (This should include details of the risks which the equipment is intended to combat, why and how it is to be used, and what the employee must do to maintain it in an efficient state. Most items needed in schools will require only basic instructions.) Employers must take all reasonable steps to ensure that equipment provided is properly used.

Employees are required to use personal protective equipment issued to them according to the instructions and training given by the employer, and to take all reasonable steps to ensure that it is returned to the storage provided after use. They must report immediately any loss of or obvious defect in the equipment.

Compliance with European directives aimed at harmonisation of standards throughout the common market area requires the adoption of European standards for the design and manufacture of most items of personal protective equipment. All personal protective equipment sold in the EEC from 1 January 1994 must have been subject to independent inspection and have been granted a certificate of conformity. Such items will bear a "CE" mark. Any equipment currently in use may continue to be used so long as it remains suitable for the purpose in question.

Application in schools

These regulations, while applying to trainees and pupils on work experience, do not apply to pupils or voluntary helpers in schools. However, the general requirements of s.3, Health and Safety at Work Act, together with the common law duty of care, will require the use of personal protective equipment by pupils in circumstances where provision for employees would be a specific legal requirement.

Some activities in schools are excluded from these regulations by virtue of being subject to other legislation (see "COSHH and Schools") but they will apply and provision may be necessary in areas such as:

(a) eye protection in CDT workshops (see "Eye Protection")
(b) life jackets for persons engaged in water sports
(c) riding helmets
(d) waterproof clothing to protect grounds staff against inclement weather
(e) gloves for gardeners
(f) special jackets, gloves, trousers and boots for grounds staff using chainsaws
(g) protection against molten metal in foundry work.

Regulation 6 requires employers to have an assessment made to ensure that any personal protective equipment that is to be provided is suitable. This follows on from the requirements of the Management of Health and Safety at Work Regulations (MHSWR) 1992 to identify hazards and evaluate the extent of the risks arising. It is sensible when employing a "competent person" to carry out MHSWR assessments to ask them also to assess the suitability (as defined by this regulation) of personal protective equipment currently in use, advise on any change in specification that may be needed and to identify any other areas where such equipment should be provided.

Further reading

Personal protective equipment at work (Regulation and Guidance Notes) L25, HSE 1992, HMSO

Electrical Safety

Over recent years schools have come to rely more and more on electricity. The increasing use of computers, televisions and audio visual aid equipment in the curricular areas has been mirrored by the increased use of electrically powered equipment in school offices and kitchens, and for cleaning and gardening operations. Whilst electricity makes a considerable contribution to most aspects of school life it also has the potential to kill and to cause fires. To enjoy the benefits without risks requires that both the school's electrical supply installation and the equipment are well designed and constructed, carefully maintained and sensibly used.

Electrical shock

In the simplest terms, the human body will act as an electrical conductor with a resistance that varies according to skin resistance. This can be as high as 100,000 ohms for dry, thick calloused skin to 1000 ohms for wet normal skin. In a shock situation a current, the magnitude of which is determined by Ohm's Law (current in amps equals the voltage divided by the resistance), flows through the body. A tingling sensation is felt at 1 mA (1 milli Amp or .001 Amp) and at 10 mA the average adult experiences muscle contractions that prevent movement of the hand/forearm. If the path of the current is across the chest and the current reaches about 30 mA the chest muscles become contracted and breathing ceases. Unless the current is switched off within two or three minutes, when breathing will restart, death occurs. In some cases, where a low to medium current passes through the chest for a short period of time, the heart goes into a condition called ventricular fibrillation, and regular heart action ceases. Even if the current is quickly removed the heart will not restart spontaneously and death occurs unless cardiac massage is immediately applied.

In a shock situation the initial resistance of the skin may limit the current but the skin resistance will quickly drop, firstly because of sweating and secondly due to carbonising of the skin. Protection against electrical shock requires:

(a) Prevention of contact with voltages that could cause a significant current flow by effective insulation.
(b) The effective earthing of all exposed metalwork so that in a fault condition fuses blow, disconnecting the supply, rather than the metal becoming live. This in turn relies on an efficient earthing system throughout the building.
(c) Where there remains a foreseeable risk the provision of devices capable of automatically and almost instantaneously switching off the supply in an accident situation.
(d) Not working on live equipment and circuits, but where this is unavoidable, ensuring that all possible protective measures are employed, that the worker is highly competent and that other persons are immediately available to give assistance in an emergency.

The Electricity at Work Regulations 1989

The Electricity at Work Regulations 1989 apply to school premises. They place a duty on employers to ensure, so far as is reasonably practicable, that an electrical installation and all electrical equipment is constructed, maintained and used so as to prevent danger. Regulations 14 and 16 prohibit working on live circuits unless it is reasonable to do so and unless suitable precautions have been taken to prevent injury and also require that persons so doing must have sufficient knowledge to prevent danger or be under competent supervision.

Guidance Note GS 23

Following the introduction of the Electricity at Work Regulations the Health and Safety Executive has issued a revised edition of Guidance Note GS 23 *Electrical Safety in Schools*, originally published in 1983. The new guidance note is essential reading for anyone responsible for electrical safety in schools. The advice given includes the following points:

(a) The fixed electrical circuits, etc within the school should be inspected and tested at least every five years by a competent person.
(b) Where wiring is subject to damage and abuse (eg surface wiring in

temporary classrooms) and in external areas such as greenhouses it should be similarly inspected every three years.

(c) Any additions or changes to the school's wiring must be inspected and tested by a competent person before power is applied. (The prosecution of an LEA and a teacher in 1989 for allowing a pupil to do such work and then not having it checked is mentioned in the guidance note.)

(d) The electrical circuits associated with stages/theatre halls should be inspected annually.

(e) Schools should keep a register of all electrical equipment and it should not be possible for apparatus previously discarded as defective to slip back into use.

(f) Equipment which was not manufactured to current standards may require modification (eg pottery kilns with exposed elements that can be touched).

(g) Home-made or modified equipment should be inspected and tested by a competent person before use.

(h) All electrical equipment operating at over 50 volts should be visually checked each term and any defective items rectified.

(i) Any hand-held equipment that has an exposed metal case should be inspected and tested by a competent person each year. (Details of the necessary testing, etc is given in the appendix.)

(j) Any double insulated equipment (ie no exposed metal casing) should be visually inspected for any damage to the insulation of the item, cable sheath or plug each time it is used.

(k) Where equipment is used outside the building via a flexible cable a residual current device (RCD) should be used in the supply circuit. (RCDs work by sensing any difference in the current flowing in the two power supply lines. If, because of an insulation failure, damage, etc an additional current flows to earth from either line, possibly via a person, the power is switched off in a fraction of a second. The trip sensitivity is predetermined; up to 30 mA will provide protection against electrical shock to earth. RCDs do not, however, provide any protection against a shock caused by connection between live and neutral.)

(l) Detailed advice is given about the use of voltages in excess of 25 volts in curricular activities.

(m) Reference is made to the need to refer to advice given in booklet HS(G)13 *Safety in Electrical Testing* for details of the precautions necessary where teachers or technicians repair or calibrate equipment such that parts live at more than 50 volts are exposed.

The guidance note defines a competent person as someone with "sufficient technical knowledge, experience and skills to be able to carry out the specific task and prevent danger or injury arising during the course of the work, or as a result of the work".

Further advice

When purchasing items of electrical equipment schools may wish to specify that they are supplied with the mains plug properly fitted and with the appropriate value of fuse installed. Plugs should only be fitted by a competent person, as defined above. It is particularly important that the plugs used are of good quality and, although they are normally supplied with a 13 ampere fuse, that a value of fuse appropriate to the equipment is used. The devices used to grip the sheath of the cable in the plug and in the equipment must be effective and equipment should not be used if it is possible to see the colour coded inner conductors of the cable. Damage to the cable sheath must not be repaired by taping, etc. If pieces break off plugs, socket outlet plates, etc they should not be used until the defective part has been replaced.

Particular care must be exercised when privately owned electrical equipment, and especially guitar amplifiers and electric guitars, are used on school premises. Inadequate earthing can produce a lethal situation. Such equipment should ideally be checked by a competent person before its use is permitted but if this is not possible it should be operated via a 1:1 isolating transformer or on a circuit protected by an RCD.

Electrical accidents

Electrical accidents in schools can sometimes be dramatic. In one case a technician overcame the problem of fuses blowing when home made photographic lights were in use by putting a copper nail in the fuse board. He touched a defective light and an earth and was lucky enough to be revived by a bystander. In two separate incidents the leader of a visiting pop group and a pupil at a boarding school were rendered unconscious when they touched earthed objects when using electric guitars. A cleaner suffered severe burns to the palm of her hand, subsequently requiring skin grafts, when she handled a taped repair to the cable of a floor scrubbing machine.

The HSE has published a summary of the electrical accidents in schools investigated by inspectors in the five years up to 1989. Thirty-nine per cent involved plugs, sockets and cables, 26 per cent involved equipment, of which over a third were floor scrubbers and buffers, 5 per cent involved stage lighting and 7 per cent science experiments.

Further reading

The Electricity at Work Regulations 1989, SI 635, HMSO
Electrical Safety in Schools, Guidance Note GS23, HSE 1990, HMSO
Electrical Safety at Places of Entertainment, Guidance Note GS50, HSE 1991, HMSO
Electrical Safety for Entertainers, 1991, HSE
Protection Against Electric Shock, Guidance Note GS27, HSE 1984, HMSO
Safety in Science Laboratories, DES 1978, HMSO
The Safe Use of Portable Electrical Apparatus (Electrical Safety), Guidance Note PM32 (REV) 1990, HMSO
Safety in Electrical Testing, Guidance Note HS(G) 13, HSE 1980
A Guide to the Electricity at Work Regulations 1989—An Open Learning Course, HMSO 1990

Woodworking Machines

It is not possible for a hand fed woodworking machine fully to comply with the general legal requirement that all dangerous parts of a machine must be guarded and for it to remain usable. The Woodworking Machines Regulations 1974 are in effect an exemption to that strict guarding requirement but they compensate for the hazards permitted to remain by spelling out conditions of use. Persons are only allowed to use circular saws, planes, thicknessers, etc if they have been sufficiently trained. The training must cover the type of work envisaged on the machine in question. It must cover the dangers arising from the use of the machine and all necessary precautions such as the methods of using guards, devices and appliances that enable machining to be carried out safely. The operative is legally responsible for the correct adjustment and use of guards, etc.

From 1 January 1993 parts of the Woodworking Machines Regulations have been replaced by the Provision and Use of Work Equipment

Regulations 1992 (PUWER) but the detailed and specific training requirements have not been repealed. The new legislation requires that machines are used only for their intended purpose (which means, for example, that circular saws must not be used for rebating work), their use is to be restricted to designated persons who are adequately trained, and supervisors must be given sufficient training to enable them to supervise the use of machines. (For full details of these requirements see Regulations 5–9, the Provisions and Use of Work Equipment Regulations 1992. Regulations 11–24, which deal with matters such as guarding, controls and maintenance apply to new equipment immediately and to existing equipment on 1 January 1997.)

In secondary schools serious injuries (amputations, severe lacerations, etc) have been suffered by staff usually because the person has not been adequately trained and occasionally because training has been ignored. One large education authority only stopped a sequence of such accidents by introducing a system of training with an assessment of competence prior to the granting of authority to use such machines. Grim experience indicates that it is necessary to ensure (by key switches or padlocks) that unauthorised persons cannot use the machines. Heads of department, craft teachers, science technicians and persons such as those using a workshop for evening classes must be prevented from putting themselves at risk, as must caretakers during weekends and holiday periods.

A notice should be fixed adjacent to each circular saw, planer, thicknesser, etc specifying by name who is designated as a user of the machine.

Woodworking machines are often crammed into small areas and this causes additional hazards. There should be a space of one metre more than the maximum length of material to be machined on three sides of the machine. If space is restricted this will mean that the maximum dimensions of material must be limited and it may be necessary, for example, for sheets of material to be cut in half by hand before machining.

Workshops housing machines must have a sound, level floor with reasonable non-slip qualities. The floor must be kept free of sawdust, chips, etc and material must not be stacked where it could cause tripping. There must be adequate lighting (see "Lighting") and a reasonable temperature must be maintained (see "Temperatures").

Except for hand-held machines, woodworking machines must be securely fixed to a floor or bench when in use. Machines should be provided with overload trip and no voltage release facilities. "Start" buttons should be recessed to prevent inadvertent operation while the "stop" buttons should be larger and mushroom headed.

Any machines in areas accessible to pupils must be additionally protected. Panels and doors that give access for adjustment and maintenance must be either locked or be fixed with a bolt that requires a special tool to release it (eg an Allen key). Fail safe micro-switches must be fitted to panels giving access to belts for speed changing on wood lathes, but because of the long run down time of the blade, micro-switches alone do not provide sufficient protection for side panels on band saws.

The DES recommends that pupils should not be allowed to use circular saws, planing machines, etc.

(See also "Control of Substances Hazardous to Health" for an example of a hazard assessment for wood dusts, and "Eye Protection".)

Further reading

Safety in the Use of Woodworking Machines, HSW 41, HMSO 1970
A Guide to the Woodworking Machines Regulations 1974, HS(R)9, HMSO
Health and Safety in Workshops of Schools and Similar Establishments BS, 4163:1984, British Standards Institution
Safety in Practical Studies, Booklet no. 3 (rev 1985) DES, HMSO
Training of Woodworking Machinists, HSE 1992, HMSO

Storage of Hazardous Materials

A number of potentially hazardous substances are found in schools. The range includes solvents, fuels, compressed gases, cleaning materials, pesticides and herbicides, and laboratory chemicals. In addition to risks such as fire, explosion and the release of toxic fumes, the possibility of interference by pupils must always be borne in mind.

Under the Packaging and Labelling of Dangerous Substances Regulations 1978, substances that are toxic, corrosive, harmful, highly flammable, irritant, explosive or oxidising must be supplied with labels specifying the hazard in words and/or symbols. The labels may also give advice on storage. If chemicals and other materials are transferred to other containers any warning labels on the original packaging must also be transferred. Soft drink containers must, of course, never be used for such purposes. Manufacturers and suppliers of substances for use at a workplace are required (s.6 HASAWA) to provide adequate information to permit the safe use of a product and this should include any special requirements for storage.

Highly flammable liquids and petrol

In addition to petrol and methylated spirits (widely used in spirit duplicators), there may be various adhesives, solvents, paints, etc which have a flashpoint below 32°C and these must be stored and used with equal care.

The type of storage required will depend on the quantity to be kept. In primary schools, and in separate departments in secondary schools where the volume to be stored does not exceed 50 litres, a metal, flame resisting cupboard may be employed. Quantities not in excess of 500 cm³ (0.5l) may be left in workrooms overnight provided that the material is in an unbreakable, stoppered container.

Larger quantities must be stored in external steel bins or in brick built stores. The advice of the local fire brigade should be obtained about the siting of such stores.

Cupboards, bins or stores containing highly flammable liquids or petrol must be marked with two signs complying with the requirements of the Safety Signs Regulations 1980. These are:

(a) a triangular warning sign with a flame pictogram in black on a yellow background (the word "flammable" should appear below the triangle)

(b) a pictogram of a cigarette and a match inside a red circle with a red diagonal bar (the words "no smoking, no naked lights" should appear below).

Such stores must also be kept locked.

The storage of more than a small quantity of petrol is subject to licensing requirements, which include the specification for the design and construction of the store. The advice of the local fire brigade should be obtained in the first instance.

Compressed gases

Cylinders containing oxygen, acetylene, liquid petroleum gas (LPG) and laboratory gases are used on school premises.

The main risk associated with gas cylinders is that of explosion. This may be caused by the application of heat (such as in a fire) or by an impact due to being dropped or falling over. There is also always a risk of leakage. Storage arrangements must be made with these possibilities in mind. A means of supporting cylinders in a vertical position must be provided unless they are kept on purpose made trolleys. The ventilation in the storage area must be sufficient to prevent a build up of flammable, toxic or asphyxiant gas in the event of a leak. Storage must be in an area where there are no combustible materials, out of direct sunlight and away from heaters, hot water pipes, etc. The fire resistance of the storage area must be such as to allow safe evacuation of the premises before a fire could affect the area.

Depending on the quantity of cylinders and the types of gas used, three kinds of storage are used in schools:

(a) A designated area, which is an identified location, perhaps in a chemical store or preparation room, to which cylinders are returned when not in use. Some means of securing the cylinders in a vertical position is required. No more than four 40 cu ft cylinders should be stored in this way.

(b) A ventilated store room: ventilation should be provided at high and low level on two walls. If flammable gases are to be stored, flameproof lighting may be required. A means of supporting cylinders in a vertical position is required. The advice of the local fire brigade should be sought prior to setting up a store of this type.

(c) An external store constructed of weld mesh on a rigid frame with a lightweight plastic roof. This type of store should be located on a north facing wall and be provided with a strong entry gate and lock, and means to secure the cylinders in an upright position.

Care must be taken to provide the maximum possible separation between flammable gases and oxygen.

Gas cylinder stores and storage areas must be provided with warning signs complying with the Safety Signs Regulations 1980. In all cases there must be a yellow sign with a black triangle containing an exclamation mark, and with the words "Compressed gases—no entry to unauthorised persons" beneath. Where any of the stored gases are flammable there must also be a "no smoking: no naked lights" sign as described above for flammable liquids stores.

Chemicals and other materials

Perhaps the most important aspect of safe storage of chemicals in science departments and similar materials in art, CDT, etc areas is stock control. Apart from the safety advantages of keeping only the minimum quantities needed, the avoidance of waste because of deterioration can represent a worthwhile saving in cash terms.

Stores should be dry, sufficiently well ventilated to deal with any fumes and vapours that may be emitted, secure and well lit. Good ventilation is particularly important where the storage area is also a workroom (eg a science preparation room). Where materials are stored above shoulder height, steps, etc should be provided to allow safe access. Large containers, such as Winchester quarts, should be stored at low level. (Sufficient Winchester carriers should be available in the store.)

Incompatible chemicals should be separated as far as it is practicable to do so (ie oxidising agents and combustibles, strong acids and strong alkalis, water reactive chemicals and aqueous solutions).

(Very detailed advice on chemical storage is given in CLEAPSS Report L148a, available to subscribers. Guidance is also given in *Safety in Science Laboratories*, DES booklet.)

Further reading

Storage and Use of Highly Flammable Liquids in Educational Establishments, HSE 1986
Substances For Use at Work: the Provision of Information, HMSO 1985
The Keeping of LPG in Cylinders and Similar Containers. Guidance Note, HMSO 1986
Do You Work with Chemicals and Other Materials in Educational Establishments? HSE 1986

Glass Accidents

Glass that would be considered to be satisfactory in domestic situations is not adequate for use in schools. A judge made this point many years ago when awarding damages to an injured pupil, but today the vast majority of glass in schools is still of the annealed type.

Accidents involving glass represent the most likely way that permanent damage will be suffered by pupils. They are also readily preventable and often at no long term cost. When a limb is thrust through a pane of glass there is often nerve damage. Modern micro-surgery can sometimes repair such damage, but not always.

Georgian wired glass is only ordinary annealed glass with wires incorporated to maintain its integrity in a fire. In an accident situation the broken pieces of glass do not fall away and terrible injuries can result. In one case a pupil who kicked a wired glass panel in a door had a 12 inch long flap of flesh from his thigh hanging down below his knee. Pupils who collide face first with wired glass panels may well suffer serious scarring.

The vast majority of glass accidents do not cause injury, of course, but reglazing does cost money. Any pane of glass that is in a vulnerable location in a school is likely to be broken sooner or later, and some panes are repeatedly broken. If annealed glass is replaced with toughened glass, long term maintenance costs will be significantly reduced, quite apart from protecting people from injury. Unfortunately, toughened glass cannot be cut to size on site but the cost becomes more reasonable if a large number of panes are ordered at the same time. An alternative medium term answer is provided by plastic films which, when applied to existing glass, significantly increase its strength. These are not unduly expensive. Where smoke stop doors with wired glass panels are concerned, plastic film is the only option at the moment. The Secretary of State for Education has powers under the Buildings Act to vary the specification of smoke stop doors but has not done so. In a recent four year period 45 people were injured in Inner London Education Authority (ILEA) schools alone due to the use of wired glass panels in smoke stop doors.

It is unfortunate that it is possible to comply with the Approved Code of Practice (ACOP) accompanying the Workplace (Health, Safety and Welfare) Regulations 1992 in respect of glazing and yet not significantly reduce the potential for pupil accidents. This may be excused by the peculiarities of the statutory accident reporting system for pupils which requires only glass accidents resulting in immediate admission to hospital for 24 hours to be reported to the Health and Safety Executive.

It is recommended that when considering the options given in the ACOP in respect of Regulation 14 annealed glass is not considered a "safety material", that the maximum height of windows requiring safety material because of a foreseeable risk of collision should be "pupil head" rather than waist height and panes should only be disregarded if narrower than 150 mm. It is an interesting thought that the pane involved in the gruesome accident described above would have complied fully with the ACOP.

Playground Safety

Over one half of all injuries to children occurring at school happen in the playground. Approximately 15 per cent of these involve collisions with buildings, 10 per cent with other pupils, 9 per cent playground games (eg *ad hoc* games of cricket, football) and 55 per cent are due to slips, trips and falls. Sixty-six per cent of serious injuries involve the upper limbs, 16 per cent the lower limbs, 9 per cent the head and 8 per cent the trunk. These figures are based on accident reports collected by ILEA between 1985 and 1989 covering approximately 300,000 pupils in nursery, primary and secondary schools.

Pupils, of course, have to be given the opportunity to let off steam, and it is better from a safety viewpoint for this to happen in the playground rather than within the school building, provided that playgrounds are reasonably safe and adequately supervised. A proportion of the accidents occurring when pupils collide with buildings are due to overcrowding and poor design (eg open windows intruding into play areas). While it is usually impossible, particularly in inner city areas, to increase the size of playgrounds, where overcrowding is a particular problem staggering break times might be considered. Hazards caused by building design can sometimes be minimised by using barriers or flower beds to keep pupils away from them but it is important not simply to exchange one problem for another (eg free standing concrete flower tubs introduced for this purpose can cause many collision type accidents).

Footballs, bats, etc used in crowded areas frequently cause injuries, usually to people not involved in the game. Where size and layout permits, such games should be restricted to one area of the playground. The use of lightweight balls is likely to reduce such problems but would be extremely unpopular with the pupils!

The surface of playgrounds should be kept in good condition and any uneven paving slabs or drain covers must be corrected. So far as it is possible, pupils should be kept away from steps, steep slopes and sudden changes in level.

Most ILEA primary and nursery schools were provided with fixed play equipment. It was estimated that 1.7 million "pupil play sessions" took place each year. The equipment was designed to BS 5696 which means, among other things, that it should not be possible to fall more than two metres in an accident. Approximately 3 per cent of all accidents in playgrounds were falls from play equipment, 85 per cent of serious injuries so caused being broken arms and collar bones, 4 per cent were to the leg and 4 per cent (or approximately one per year) to the head.

This breakdown is interesting because governors, LEAs and schools are often pressed by anxious parents to provide "safety" surfaces beneath play equipment. These surfaces are expensive to install and do not have an unlimited life. They will certainly reduce the severity of head injuries caused by striking the ground. However, over 95 per cent of serious injuries arising from the use of play equipment are caused by falling awkwardly or striking equipment or other pupils, and most safety surfaces have no effect in these cases. The ILEA statistics suggest that even with intensive usage, each set of play equipment will cause a serious head injury once in about 400 years. If it is decided to install a safety surface it is important to remember that the area does not become "safe" and there will continue to be a need to consider the following points if serious injuries are to be avoided:

(a) the equipment must be well designed, sensibly sited, correctly installed and well maintained
(b) the equipment must be appropriate for the age, strength and abilities of the pupils using it
(c) the use of equipment must always be adequately supervised and dangerous behaviour prevented
(d) only children of similar size and abilities should use the equipment at any one time.

If it is decided to provide an impact absorbing surface below play equipment various materials are available. Organisations in Sweden, Australia, Canada and Holland have compared the shock absorbing characteristics of such materials and their results suggest that pea shingle, sand and woodchips or bark are two to three times more effective than grass or rubber surfaces, which in turn are about one and one half times more effective than is ashphalt.

Woodbark or chips (preferably from conifers), is inexpensive, has high impact absorbing qualities, is easy to maintain, has a reasonable life expectancy and may reduce the incidence of fractures caused by awkward falls. It is necessary to exclude dogs and cats from the material to prevent fouling, so the initial cost may be increased by the need to provide fencing. It requires a daily check for cleanliness and depth (300 mm is usual), and regular raking and levelling. Where these requirements can be met this material is probably the best choice.

Further reading

King, K and Ball, D *A Holistic Approach to Accident and Injury Prevention in Children's Playgrounds*, LSS 1989 (Available from LSS, Great Guildford House, Great Guildford Street, London SE1 0ES)
Play Equipment Intended for Permanent Installation Outdoors, BS 5696, British Standards Institution 1978

Swimming Pools

The safe maintenance of swimming pools requires attention to detail, care in the handling, storage and use of chemicals and an appreciation of the importance of water quality control.

Disinfection systems

The vast majority of school swimming pools use chlorine to disinfect the water. Chlorine is a gas with a pungent bleach smell and a greenish-yellow colour. It is highly irritant to the lungs and can cause death. Incidents occur from time to time when an error in the handling of pool chemicals allows the release of chlorine. Breathing chlorine gas can produce effects that are delayed for up to 24 hours so an accidental release often results in numbers of pupils and staff being detained in hospital for observation.

The most common systems employ either sodium hypochlorite or trichloroisocyanuric acid.

Ten per cent—14 per cent hypochlorite is added to the pool water either directly or, more usually, by being bled into a flow and return dosing arrangement. This tends to make the water alkaline which, unless corrected, causes it to become cloudy and reduces the efficiency of the disinfection process. (Efficient disinfection requires 2ppm—3ppm of free chlorine and a water pH between 7.5 to 8.0, but ideally between 7.6 and 7.8.) Hydrochloric acid (5 per cent) is added to the water to maintain the correct pH level. If the sodium hypochlorite and hydrochloric acid solutions are directly mixed, quantities of chlorine gas are immediately generated. All necessary precautions must be taken to avoid this happening. The chemicals must be stored separately. A colour coding system is normally used to reduce the chance of a chemical being added to the wrong dosing tank, and the two tanks are usually physically separated, with bunds to prevent mixing should a spillage or leakage occur.

Trichloroisocyanuric acid is supplied in tablet form. The tablets are dosed into the water via a special apparatus. This chemical tends to make the water acidic and soda ash is periodically added to maintain the optimum pH value. Chlorine is released when the tablets come into contact with water. There is also a small release in store, and the storage area must be dry and with good low level ventilation.

Swimming pool installations should only be operated by trained persons. Dosing should never be carried out while the pool is in use or the area is occupied. The plant room must be kept locked and admittance to unauthorised persons prohibited.

Protective clothing must be worn when handling pool chemicals when there is any risk of splashing or other contamination. Goggles or face shield to BS2092 'C', waterproof apron, rubber gloves and rubber boots must be provided. When filling tablet dosing units, a canister respirator giving protection against chlorine must be worn.

Water quality

The quality of pool water depends on the capacity and efficiency of the purification system and the number of bathers using the pool. If a pool is over-used the water will be inadequately treated and there will be a risk of the spread of disease. Infections such as typhoid, dysentery, gastroenteritis and poliomyelitis can be transmitted in this way. Ear and eye infections and "swimming pool itch" may occur if dosing is incorrect. Sore eyes are blamed on too much chlorine in the water but in practice the cause is often insufficient chlorine. In clearing the water the chlorine combines with ammonia type chemicals, forming chloramines. It is these that produce sore eyes and itching.

Further reading

The Treatment and Quality of Swimming Pool Water, Department of the Environment, HMSO 1985
Swimming Pool Disinfection Systems Using Sodium Hypochlorite, Guidelines for Design and Operation, Department of the Environment, HMSO 1979

Swimming Pool Disinfection Systems Using Calcium Hypochlorite, Chloroiso-cyanurates, Halogenated Dimethythydantoins and Solid Ancillary Chemicals, Guidelines for Design and Operation, Department of the Environment, HMSO 1981
Safety in Swimming Pools, Sports Council 1988

Work with Glass Reinforced Plastics

The main hazard arising from glass reinforced plastics (GRP) fabrication is the exposure of users to styrene. In 1978 a prohibition notice was served on the Inner London Education Authority (ILEA) following the discovery by an inspector of a person using this material in the repair of the inside of a canoe. Styrene is heavier than air and very high levels were found to have collected inside the hull. The approach that the ILEA adopted makes an interesting study because it shows that problems can be solved without large expenditure. To overcome the problem with canoe repairs involved putting a flexible extraction hose inside the craft so that clean air was continuously drawn in past the person's breathing zone. The greatest difficulty, however, was that the notice was worded "fibreglass repair inside boats or similar work involving the emission of styrene in confined spaces", and it therefore applied to GRP work in various forms being carried on at over 100 different locations on ILEA premises. While being anxious to avoid banning a curricular activity it would have been enormously expensive to provide mechanical extraction systems at all of those places, and quite unjustifiable considering that the work was typically only carried on for two weeks per year.

A series of experiments were carried out in order to determine the maximum quantity of material that could be used in a standard sized classroom without exceeding a level of 25 per cent of the legal limit for exposure. The following conditions for use were published, implemented and periodically monitored:

(a) work could only take place out of doors or indoors in rooms with a floor area in excess of 89 square metres
(b) work would be timetabled to take place in the summer months so that all windows could be kept open
(c) maximum total quantity of material, either being laid up or curing, to be in the room at any one time would not exceed one square metre
(d) work would only be carried out at bench level.

Engineering Inspections

Prior to the Health and Safety at Work, etc Act 1974 (HASAWA) there were a number of requirements in various statutory provisions for the formal periodic inspection of certain plant and equipment by "competent persons". These requirements had been introduced over a 75 year period, usually in response to catastrophic failures caused by unnoticed wear, tear and deterioration.

S.2(a) HASAWA lays a duty on employers that requires the "provision and maintenance of plant and systems of work that are, so far as is reasonably practicable, safe and without risks to health". While most of the previous legislation did not apply to schools it provides a valuable indication of what is necessary to discharge the duties arising from s.2(a). Regulations made under HASAWA, and therefore directly applying to schools, have extended the requirements for inspections by "competent persons" (see "Electrical Safety" and "Control of Substances Hazardous to Health" (COSHH)).

"Competent persons"

Although the various statutes specify that engineering inspections are to be carried out by competent persons they provide little guidance as to what the term actually means. Health and Safety Executive Guidance Note GS 23 *Electrical Safety in Schools* gives a definition but qualifies it by saying that it is "for the purposes of this guidance note". The definition is, however, as good as any. It says that "a competent person is a person who possesses sufficient technical knowledge, experience and skills to be able to carry out the specific task and prevent danger or injury arising during the course of the work or as a result of the work".

Specialist engineering insurance companies have long employed engineer surveyors who act as competent persons, carrying out inspections on steam boilers, cranes, lifts, etc.

For the periodic inspection of gas installations and appliances members of the Confederation of Registered Gas Installers (CORGI) would be considered "competent".

The periodic inspection of fume cupboards could be carried out by persons such as technicians provided that they have received adequate training.

Some LEAs employ engineers, electricians, etc to carry out engineering inspections in their schools.

Plant and equipment in schools

Plant and equipment in schools that should be subject to periodic inspection include:

(a) lifts, including manually operated food and goods lifts

(b) cradles and associated equipment used for window cleaning, etc

(c) fume cupboards, dust collection facilities and mechanical ventilation systems provided to protect persons using hazardous substances (see "Control of Substances Hazardous to Health")

(d) the electrical supply installation and electrical equipment (see "Electrical Safety")

(e) gas supply pipework, controls and appliances

(f) fixed PE apparatus

(g) ropes, hawsers, pulleys, etc used in areas such as halls, stage areas

(h) eyebolts provided to safeguard persons cleaning windows

(i) boilers

(j) autoclaves and pressure cookers

(k) hoists used in conjunction with lifting beams in laboratories.

In all cases formal records must be kept of such inspections.

Further reading

Guidance Notes on Gas Safety in Educational Establishments, DES and British Gas plc, Service Engineering, 326 High Holborn, London WC1V 7PT.

Offices, Shops and Railway Premises (Hoists and Lifts) Regulations 1968, HMSO

Guidance Note: Electrical Safety in Schools (Electricity at Work) Regulations 1989, GS23 HSE, HMSO

Maintenance of Mechanical Services, Architects and Building Branch Bulletin 70, DES 1990, HMSO

A Guide to the Pressure System and Transportable Gas Containers Regulations 1989, Guidance Document, HMSO

Fume Cupboards in Schools, DES Design Note 29, 1982

Danger: Gas Appliances, IND(G) 79(L) REV, HSE

Eye Protection

Eye protection must be worn by employees and pupils whenever there is a foreseeable risk of injury to the eyes. Failure to observe this simple requirement resulted in the first prosecution of a school teacher under the Health and Safety at Work, etc Act 1974. A head of chemistry who failed to use available safety screens or eye protectors to safeguard pupils while carrying out an experiment was convicted and fined £500.

Headteachers need to satisfy themselves that heads of practical departments have, and have effectively implemented, arrangements covering the use of eye protection. Heads of department need to take all reasonable steps to ensure that the employees for whom they are responsible are using eye protection when necessary. While this does not mean continuous supervision it does mean spot checks at intervals and suitable measures being taken if evidence of non-compliance is found. Individual employees are required to use eye protection provided to them and to report any loss of or defect in the protectors (Personal Protective Equipment at Work Regulations 1992 or, in the case of substances, Control of Substances Hazardous to Health Regulations 1988). They must also ensure that "others" (ie pupils) use eye protection as necessary (s.7 Health and Safety at Work, etc Act).

Few, if any, schools do not have some form of eye protection available for use in practical and science areas. A common failing, however, is that the type of eye protection used is not appropriate to deal with the particular hazard involved.

At the time of writing all eye protectors used in schools must be manufactured to BS 2092, except for those used for welding, etc, where they must conform to BS 1542. A marking system is used to indicate the level and type of protection provided by a device:

BS 2092   – low impact, general purpose
BS 2092.2   – medium impact, general purpose
BS 2092.1   – high impact, general purpose
BS 2092.1M   – high impact, general purpose and protection against molten metal

Similarly "C" indicates protection against chemical splash and dust, "D" dust resistance and "G" gas tight qualities. However harmonisation of standards throughout Europe means that BS 2092 will shortly be replaced by BS EN 166, 167 and 168. All eye potection sold in the EC from 1

January 1994 will have to have been granted a certificate of conformity and bear a "CE" mark. Eye protectors in use before that date may continue to be used so long as they remain suitable for the purpose in question (see Personal Protective Equipment at Work Regulations 1992).

The following three kinds of eye protector are generally used in schools.

Safety spectacles

Low impact, general purpose devices. These do not provide complete protection against chemical splashes, dusts or molten metal. They are, however, comfortable to wear for long periods.

Safety spectacles provide adequate protection when handling substances which are of only moderate hazard (ie not alkali solutions of molar strength or greater, concentrated acids, corrosive solids, bromine or toxic chemicals) or for stretching metal wires or plastic cords, glass working and dissection work, etc.

(Eye injuries regularly occur when hot slag is chipped from welds because the face shield is, of course, discarded as soon as the arc is extinguished. It is recommended that safety spectacles be worn in addition to using the face shield.)

Goggles

These are available with high impact, molten metal, chemical splash, dust and gas resisting qualities. Goggles are available which give protection against a range of hazards (eg "BS 2092.1 MCD"), thus avoiding the need to have several different types for different activities. Goggles are less comfortable to wear, particularly for wearers of spectacles. (Goggles designed to be worn over spectacles are available.)

Goggles designated "BS 2092.1 MCD" will provide adequate protection for the following activities:

(a) lathe work (wood and metal)
(b) pickling
(c) etching
(d) enamelling
(e) use of resins and liquid plastics
(f) glass blowing and working
(g) hot and cold riveting
(h) forging

(i) fettling

(j) wood sanding by machine

(k) sculpting stone, etc

(l) grinding

(m) brisking

(n) buffing

(o) spot welding and metal machining

(p) working under motor vehicles.

Goggles designated impact 1, plus metal splash with an appropriate filter, should be used for gas welding and cutting.

Goggles marked "BS 2092 C" give adequate protection when handling strong alkali solutions, concentrated acids (including Millon's reagent, bromine, corrosive solids and substances labelled with a skull and cross-bones).

Full face shields

These protect the whole face as well as the eyes. Their use is required in electric arc welding, foundry work, when dispensing large volumes of concentrated acids, alkalis or other corrosive substances, when opening and dispensing containers which may be under pressure (eg silicon tetra chloride or "880" ammonia), and when handling molten alkalis.

Each member of staff who is regularly required to use eye protection should be given a personal issue of appropriate devices. Employers may not make a charge for such issues. Where an employee needs to wear safety spectacles for a number of hours per week but in practice has to wear goggles over prescription spectacles the employer should consider providing prescription safety spectacles.

Personal issue of face shields and specialised goggles (eg for welding) are unlikely to be warranted but they must be available within the work area as required.

General

Sufficient class sets of protectors must be available for use by pupils. Each set should include a proportion of goggles designed to be worn over spectacles. There does not appear to be any evidence supporting fears that infections such as conjunctivitis could be spread by the use of communal eye protectors, and the London School of Hygiene and Tropical Medicine has stated that viable lice are not transmitted by headwear.

Eye protectors should be washed with washing up liquid every few weeks. They may be disinfected by immersion in a weak solution of Dettol or Centrimide. They should be thoroughly rinsed and dried carefully to avoid scratching, and then inspected for damage and optical clarity. (Replacement lenses are available for some devices.)

It must be remembered that persons in the vicinity of a work activity may be just as much at risk of injury to the eyes as the person directly involved. When a potentially hazardous operation is demonstrated, close observers must be adequately protected and sufficient spare eye protectors must be available to equip visitors to any area where eye protection is being worn.

Stories about a contact lens being welded to someone's cornea due to exposure to an electric arc flash are completely without foundation but their use can present problems. They are difficult to remove in an emergency situation (assuming that the person attempting to give first aid knows that they are present) and the soft type may absorb chemicals and prolong contact with the cornea. Pupils should be discouraged from wearing contact lenses in practical lessons but if they do so they should wear goggles whatever the level of eye protection being worn by the other pupils.

Persons unwilling or unable to wear appropriate eye protection must not be allowed to be present in any area where a risk to the eyes exists.

In civil law there is a long established principle that precautions satisfying the duty of care towards a normally sighted person would not necessarily be considered to be adequate where a person having an existing impairment of sight is concerned. This is because the loss of an eye would be so much more serious to such a person. Where partially sighted persons are at risk it is therefore necessary to take precautions in excess of those that would normally be considered reasonable.

Eye washing

In any work area where it is foreseeable that chemicals could get into someone's eyes facilities must be provided to allow for immediate flushing. Where cold running water is available the preferred method is to provide a length of rubber tubing of a size suitable for pushing onto a tap. If running water is not available water in bottles that are specifically designed to facilitate eye flushing and to maintain the sterility of the water until it is required must be provided. Eye wash bottles must be kept in a readily available position and be regularly checked to ensure that the sterility of the contents has not been compromised.

Ladders and Steps

An all too common cause of injury in schools is the use of substitutes for ladders and steps. Chairs, tables and even chairs placed on tables are used by staff when fixing pupils' work to walls, putting up decorations at Christmas or reaching the upper shelves in the stock room. Where ladders or a pair of steps are available they are often unsuitable for the task in question or they are used in an unsafe manner.

Apart from the legal implications, not to provide suitable access equipment is a false economy. Its cost will be far outweighed by the loss for only a few days of, say, a teacher injured in a fall. Having provided suitable equipment it is important not to assume that everyone knows how to use it safely. They must be fully briefed on its limitations in use.

Stepladders

Aluminium steps that are of sound construction and of adequate length for the intended working height should be purchased. When working on a stepladder a person's waist should never be higher than the top of the steps. Some steps have treads to within a few inches of the top but this is a matter of convenience of construction rather than any intention by the designer that the upper treads should be stood on. When in use the steps should be at right angles to the work, and the stays fully extended or, where appropriate, locked down. When using steps it is important not to over-reach, and never to stand with one foot on the steps and the other on a fixed surface. If steps are to be used for access to electrical fittings operating up to 250 volts they should be equipped with insulated rubber "feet". Stepladders should only be used on a firm, solid surface.

Ladders

A ladder must be of sufficient length to allow it to be set up properly, (ie one metre out from the wall for each four metres of vertical height). When in use the ladder must either be tied at the top or an assistant must "foot" the bottom. The head of the ladder must be rested against a firm support, with both stiles making equal contact. The foot must be on firm ground, and wedges, bricks, boxes or planks must not be used to compensate for an uneven surface.

Maintenance of steps and ladders

Once per term ladders and steps should be checked for defects. If any are found the equipment should be clearly labelled "unsafe" and taken out of service. (See "Provision and Use of Work Equipment Regulations 1992".)

Safety Signs

The Safety Signs Regulations 1980 require that all safety signs in workplaces comply with British Standard 5378:1976. These regulations were introduced in response to an EC directive intended to standardise such signs throughout Europe in the interests of workers taking advantage of the increasing freedom of movement between countries.

BS 5378:1976 Part 1 divides safety signs into four categories according to the type of message. Each category has its own distinctive colour and shape. The safety colours are yellow, blue, red and green.

Stop or prohibition signs must be red, with the contrasting colour in white and any symbol in black. Cautionary or risk of danger signs must be yellow with black contrasting symbol. Safe conditions or safety are indicated by green signs with white, while blue is used for mandatory signs, again with white. BS 5378:1976 also gives 23 standard symbols for signs such as "no smoking", "first aid", and "not drinking water".

Signs erected on school access roads to control traffic must comply with the Traffic Signs Regulations and General Directions 1981 (SI 1981 No. 859) and the Highway Code as used on public highways.

Safety signs are commercially available printed on various materials, including metal sheet, rigid PVC and self-adhesive vinyl sheeting. Some types are available in a photoluminescent form and glow brightly in the dark for an hour or so after exposure to light, and these are particularly useful for escape route and exit signs.

There are a number of manufacturers of safety signs and they will provide on request coloured catalogues from which requirements can readily be selected.

Any undue proliferation of safety signs should be avoided. They should be installed only where necessary so that their impact is not diluted. Self-adhesive signs should not be used in positions accessible to pupils.

A new EC directive on safety signs was adopted in June 1992 and regulations implementing it will be made to come into effect by June 1994. The new regulations will extend existing requirements so that:

(a) *employers will be required to use a safety sign where there is a hazard that has not been adequately controlled by other means, giving due regard to assessments made under the Management of Health and Safety at Work Regulations 1992*

(b) *the number of approved safety signs will be increased and will include a number identifying fire fighting equipment*

(c) *the term "safety sign" will be extended to cover other methods of communication such as the colour coding of pipework, and acoustic signals (eg fire alarms)*

(d) *where and how safety signs should be used will be prescribed in certain cases.*

The Directive allows for a transitional period to the end of 1995 for any existing "obsolete" signs.

Further reading

Guide to the Safety Signs Regulations, HSE, HMSO
Safety Signs Catalogue, Broome Signs, 44 Buxton Road, Luton, Beds
Safety Signs Catalogue, Signs and Labels Ltd, Bradbury Industrial Park, Stockport, Cheshire, SK6 2SD

Abrasive Wheels

Machines using abrasive wheels, discs, cones, etc are similar to woodworking machines in that it is impossible to enclose totally or guard the dangerous parts and still use them for their intended purpose. The Abrasive Wheels Regulations 1970 effectively give exemption from the strict guarding requirements of the Factories Act 1961 but seek to compensate for any hazards that might arise as a consequence.

The most dangerous situation arising from the use of grinding wheels is the break up of a wheel at speed. Pieces of stone are ejected at great velocity and are capable of causing serious injury.

The regulations specify that anyone mounting an abrasive wheel on a grinding machine must have been trained, be competent and be appointed in writing. Machines must be labelled with the maximum working speed of the spindles, and wheels have either to be marked with the maximum operating speed or (for wheels less than 55 mm in diameter) the information has to be immediately to hand. A copy of Cautionary Notice F2347 should be displayed near the machine. The regulations also specify precautions to be taken in the design and support of various types of wheel, in the design and use of rests and in the provision of stop/start buttons. A schedule attached spells out the training requirements for the competent person, mentioned above. (See also "Eye Protection".)

The Abrasive Wheels Regulations 1970 will continue to operate alongside the Provision and Use of Work Equipment Regulations 1992 (PUWER) until 1 January 1997. During that period they will apply to machines which were in use at 1 January 1993. From the end of 1996 PUWER will apply in all cases and much of the old legislation will be superseded. However, the specific training requirements in the Abrasive Wheels Regulations will not be repealed.

Further reading

Safety in the Use of Abrasive Wheels, HS(G)17, HSE, HMSO 1992

Contractors on School Premises

Ideally all maintenance to school premises is carried out during holiday periods and at weekends, but in practice this does not usually prove to be possible. When contractors work on occupied school premises significant risks of injury, loss and damage are introduced which can only be controlled by careful planning and firm management.

It must be remembered that contractors need to be able to carry out their work within the time scale that they quoted for if they are not to lose financially. It is therefore important that any constraints on their operations in the interests of the school are made known to the contractor before the contract is let. Failure to do this may result in claims for increased costs.

For all but minor tasks the headteacher, contractor and, where appropriate, the architect or LEA technical officer responsible for the work, need to meet at an early stage to agree any restrictions on working that must be imposed. If cover can be arranged, safety representatives should also be invited to such meetings. Where the nature of the works allows for part of the premises to be effectively fenced off and handed over to the contractor matters are simplified to some extent, but where operations such as rewiring or decorating are carried out on occupied premises, detailed planning and subsequent regular liaison meetings with the contractor will be necessary.

The following points are among those that would need to be considered for a typical contract:

(a) Who will act as a liaison officer on behalf of the contractor during the contract?
(b) What is the name and telephone number of the supervising architect or technical officer?
(c) What will be the nature and extent of the site perimeter fencing? (A fence of two metres height is considered to be a reasonable minimum.)
(d) How and where will the contractor secure materials? (A fenced compound is necessary in most instances.)
(e) Where work areas cannot be totally isolated, what additional supervision of pupils will be necessary at class changes, break times, etc?
(f) Will the work cause problems for the school, such as noise, dust, paint fumes? (It may be necessary to agree that noisy operations are suspended at examination times, or to arrange for extra cleaning of premises. What measures can be taken to minimise such problems? Are there any indications in the data sheets provided by the manufacturers of any substances to be used of risks to the health of staff or pupils?)
(g) Scaffolding on the face of buildings provides a ready means of access for thieves and vandals. Is it necessary to secure valuable equipment or arrange for security checks by the caretaker or police in the evenings and at weekends? Is there anything that the contractor can do to help?
(h) Are there any times when operations such as the erection of scaffolds, fencing, movement of mobile scaffolds, etc should not be carried out because of pupils being in the vicinity?
(i) Is there a requirement for the screening of areas such as toilets, changing rooms and showers prior to works commencing?
(j) What precautions will be taken to prevent debris, etc falling into areas used by pupils and staff?

(k) Where and when will contractors' vehicles come onto site? Is it possible to provide a separate means of access?
(l) Will fire escape routes and means of access for fire engines be kept clear at all times?
(m) Will work in the vicinity of glazed roof lights or fragile roof coverings or the use of hot tar on roof surfaces warrant the evacuation of the areas below?
(n) If the works involve burning off external paint does the old paint contain lead? If it does, what measures will be taken to prevent lead in dust contamination of the playground?

During the progress of works it may well prove necessary to increase levels of supervision of pupils. Where minor works, such as the replacement of windows or high level electrical fittings, is being carried out detailed formal arrangements may not be warranted, but experience has shown the importance of not leaving mobile scaffolds unattended and pupils unsupervised in their vicinity. (See Regulations 8 to 10, Management of Health and Safety at Work Regulations, 1992.)

Further reading

Building Contracts on Educational Premises; Strategies for the Health and Safety of Staff and Pupils, ESAC (booklet and training package), HMSO

Chapter 11
Manual Handling

Each year about 46 million working days are lost in the United Kingdom because of back injuries and one third of all accidents reported to the Health and Safety Executive are associated with the manual handling of loads. This drain on national resources, not to mention pain and suffering, is not confined to heavy industry. It is also found in areas such as banking and retail distribution, while for health service workers manual handling accounts for over half of all injuries. In schools caretakers, kitchen workers and staff required to assist pupils with physical disabilities are particularly at risk.

In the past legislation specific to various industries was introduced to limit the maximum weight that could be lifted by a worker. This approach has proved to be ineffective. It is now recognised that a range of factors other than just weight have to be considered when seeking to minimise the risk of such injury.

The Manual Handling Operations Regulations 1992

These regulations, introduced in response to the European directive on Manual Handling, adopt a three stage approach:

(a) avoid manual handling activities involving risk, so far as is reasonably practicable, by eliminating the need to move a load or by mechanising the process
(b) where such activities involving risk cannot be avoided they should be subject to an assessment

(c) the risk of injury should be reduced, so far as is reasonably practicable.

The Management of Health and Safety at Work Regulations 1992 (MHSWR) requires employers to make a general assessment of the risks to health and safety of employees at work. Where this assessment finds that there are possible risks arising from manual handling the requirements of these regulations must be considered. (To assist the competent person carrying out the assessment to determine which activities warrant more detailed examination a system of guidelines has been provided at Appendix 1 to the Health and Safety Executive publication *Manual Handling* (see "Further Reading").)

These regulations came into force on 1 January 1993. Regulation 4(1)(a) requires that, so far as is reasonably practicable, employers will avoid the need for any manual handling operation which involves a risk of injury.

"Manual handling operation" means the lifting, movement, transporting, supporting in a static posture, and/or the intentional dropping or throwing of a "load" by human effort. (A "load" could be a human patient.) Where the MHSWR assessment indicates a possible risk of injury a preliminary judgement is made. If the risk is trivial it may be disregarded, but where this is not so consideration must be given to ways of avoiding the operation (eg could pupils collect milk from where the crates have been delivered rather than take the crates to the pupils? Is it possible to specify that deliveries of supplies to the kitchens will be made to the store room, rather than to the area outside?).

Where it is not reasonably practicable to avoid the need for employees to carry out a handling operation involving risk, Regulation 4(1)(b)(i) requires that a "suitable and sufficient" assessment be carried out.

Detailed guidance is provided on how the task, the load, the working environment and any physical requirements and the state of health of the individual concerned are to be assessed. In schools it is unlikely that anyone with the appropriate expertise will be available in-house to carry out this task and it is sensible to use the services of the "competent person" who carried out the MHSWR assessment. It is important, however, to ensure that he or she is properly briefed on the nature and extent of handling operations carried on in specialist areas, such as in schools for pupils with physical disabilities and including details of any carrying of pupils in evacuation procedures.

Regulation 4(1)(b)(ii) requires that, where it is not reasonably practicable to avoid manual handling operations which involve a risk of injury, appropriate steps must be taken to reduce that risk to the lowest level that is reasonably practicable.

Appropriate steps may include providing specific training, providing mechanical assistance such as trolleys or sack barrows, specifying that two persons must carry out a particular task, improving the layout and lighting of storerooms (heavy loads should be at waist height, lighter loads at higher or lower levels), specifying the supply of smaller sized packages (eg potatoes in 14 k rather than 25 k sacks), providing carrying devices for awkward loads such as Winchesters, and nominating particular individuals to carry out tasks that may be beyond the physical capabilities of others.

Where it is not reasonably practicable to avoid a risk arising from manual handling, Regulation 4(1)(b)(iii) requires employers to take appropriate steps to provide general and, where it is reasonably practicable to do so, precise information on the weight of each load, and on the heaviest side of a load where the centre of gravity is not central.

General information would normally be given during training or as a briefing prior to dealing with an unusual or unfamiliar load. Suppliers of items for use at work have a responsibility, under s.6 Health and Safety at Work, etc Act, for the safety of others handling their products and schools can reasonably expect that any package of significant weight should be delivered precisely marked with such, and with the centre of gravity indicated where this is offset.

Regulation 4(2) requires that employers review an assessment made under these regulations where there is reason to suspect that it is no longer valid, or where there has been a significant change in a handling operation. It must also be reviewed if a reportable injury (see "Accident Recording and Reporting") occurs as a result of a handling operation.

Employees are charged by Regulation 5 to make full and proper use of any system of work provided under Regulation 4(1)(b)(ii), above.

This makes explicit so far as manual handling operations are concerned the requirements of s.7 Health and Safety at Work, etc Act for employees to take reasonable care of themselves and others at work, and to cooperate with employers to enable them to discharge their statutory duties.

It is important to involve staff, their safety representatives and the school safety committee in the assessment process described above. The individuals carrying out tasks will know better than heads of department which represent particular difficulties.

Further reading

Manual Handling (Regulations and Guidance Notes), HSE 1992, HMSO

Chapter 12

Health, Diseases and Hygiene

Infectious Diseases

The responsibility for medical health matters on school premises is divided among various agencies. The local district health authority is responsible for all aspects of pupil health, while most LEAs have a medical officer who covers employee medical matters. School doctors (strictly school medical officers) are appointed by the district health authority, which also employs school nurses. The local authority employs a medical officer for environmental health (MOEH) and environmental health officers who have various enforcement powers in respect of certain health related issues.

Cases of some infectious diseases are notifiable and these requirements are listed in the tables on pages 135–8. Responsibility for notifying the MOEH rests with the school doctor. Following notification the school doctor and the MOEH may instruct that precautionary measures, such as the decontamination of certain areas, are implemented. Early notification is important.

Bacillary dysentery

This is an acute infection of the intestines. It is endemic in this country and is a common cause of epidemics which sweep through schools, usually in the spring and autumn terms. Nursery and primary school pupils are particularly susceptible. Transmission in schools is usually due to a lack of hand washing after using the toilet. The organisms are transferred from contaminated hands to door handles, pencils, crockery, etc and others, having touched these objects, put their hands in their mouth.

Food poisoning

Food poisoning occurs in two main ways. Food may be contaminated with toxins produced by germs (eg staphylococcal food poisoning) or by the germs themselves (eg salmonella food poisoning). Staphyloccocal cases are usually due to food being contaminated by someone suffering with an infected skin, nose or throat. The germs multiply in the food producing toxins which are not destroyed by cooking. Salmonella cases arise because of poor personal hygiene on the part of a carrier who handles food, or by a failure to cook thoroughly food which may be naturally contaminated. People suffering with salmonella poisoning produce stools that are infectious so their personal hygiene must be especially thorough if further transmission is to be avoided.

School kitchens should keep samples of all meals served in the freezer for at least 48 hours. In the event of any possible food poisoning case the samples should be made available to the environmental health officers as quickly as possible.

Gastroenteritis

This may be caused by a variety of different micro-organisms, usually entering the body with food contaminated by unhygienic handling, or by an infected person coughing or breathing on it. It may also be transmitted via inanimate objects as described above under dysentery. Outbreaks are not uncommon in nursery schools and infection tends to be more serious in effect where young children are concerned.

Hepatitis A (yellow jaundice)

This is inflammation of the liver by a virus. Transmission is, again, by eating food contaminated by someone with poor personal hygiene, by eating inadequately or uncooked food, or via inanimate objects.

Hepatitis B (serum hepatitis)

This is an uncommon virus infection causing a more severe illness than hepatitis A. The virus is carried in the blood of sufferers and transmission is by direct introduction of blood, saliva, etc into the blood stream. There is a higher than average number of carriers among mentally handicapped pupils in residential establishments and the resulting greater risk to staff working in such schools is considered by the Department of Health to warrant vaccination.

Vaccination is not considered necessary in the general school situation. Hepatitis B has a long incubation period and provided treatment is given within seven days of infection it is possible to avoid development of the disease. If, at any time, body fluids such as blood, saliva, semen, etc from another person enters a wound, cut, etc, if bites occur such that the skin is broken or if the skin is pierced by an object that has been in contact with someone else's body fluids, the victim should be advised to consult a general practitioner as soon as possible, and certainly within seven days.

Measles

This is a highly infectious disease caused by a virus. Epidemics are quite common in schools, particularly in the spring. For most children the effects are mild, and an attack gives permanent immunity, but pupils with congenital heart disease, who are delicate or who have Down's Syndrome may be at risk.

Rubella (German measles)

This is a mild virus infection that can spread rapidly in schools. (See "Pregnancy".)

Meningitis

This is a serious illness involving the irritation or infection of the membranes of the brain. It is caused by various micro-organisms which may be carried in the throat and nose of otherwise healthy people. Prompt treatment may be life saving and any possible case must be quickly referred to hospital. There is a greater risk of spread of the disease in residential establishments than in day schools.

Mumps

This is a not very infectious viral disease that causes swelling of the saliva glands. Epidemics occur every six or seven years. It is usually a mild disease with no long term ill effects but in males past puberty severe swelling of the testicles may result, with possible impairment of fertility.

Male staff who have not previously had mumps should consult their GP if they believe that they have been in contact with a case.

Chicken pox

This is a highly infectious viral disease spread by droplets exhaled by infected persons. It is mild in effect but may attack adults severely if they have not gained the immunity given by a previous infection.

Whooping cough

This disease, spread by droplets from infected persons, has largely been eliminated by mass vaccination. Cases still occur in unvaccinated children. It is a potentially serious illness for children under five.

Poliomyelitis

Occasional cases still occur among unvaccinated children. Transmission may be due to inadequate personal hygiene of a carrier, or the use of an inadequately disinfected swimming pool.

Acquired Immune Deficiency Syndrome (AIDS) and Human Immunodeficiency Virus (HIV)

AIDS is a disease which may follow infection with HIV. HIV does not spread easily and is restricted to "at risk" groups such as the sexual partners of infected people and intravenous drug misusers. HIV can only be transmitted by infected body fluids entering into someone's blood stream. It cannot be passed by normal social contacts.

Sensible hygiene precautions should be taken when dealing with cuts and spillages of body fluids (see "Hygiene"). Pupils should be warned about the hazards of forming blood brother/sisterhoods and of tattooing. Experiments in science lessons involving samples of blood must no longer be carried out. Detailed advice on dealing with possible difficulties arising from having pupils at school who are HIV positive is given in the following booklets published by the DES.

Further reading

Children at School and Problems Related to AIDS, DES 1986
AIDS: Some Questions and Answers, DES 1987

Disease	Notify		Cases – minimum period of exclusion	Contacts – necessary action
	School doctor	Medical Officer of Environmental Health		
AIDS/HIV	NO	NO		–
Chicken pox	YES	NO	Six days from onset of rash	–
Conjunctivitis	YES	NO	As advised by school doctor	–
Diphtheria	YES	YES	Until certified by school doctor	Exclude if at home. If at school, as advised by school doctor
Rubella (German measles)	YES	NO	Four days from onset of rash	See "Pregnancy"
Glandular fever	YES	NO	Until certified well	–
Influenza	YES	NO	Until recovered	–
Hepatitis A (infective hepatitis, yellow jaundice)	YES	YES	Seven days from onset of jaundice and until recovered	Consult school doctor
Hepatitis B (serum hepatitis)	YES	NO	As advised by school doctor	–

Disease	Notify		Cases – minimum period of exclusion	Contacts – necessary action
	School doctor	Medical Officer of Environmental Health		
Measles	YES	YES	Seven days from onset of rash	–
Meningitis	YES	YES	Until certified well	Consult school doctor
Mumps	YES	NO	Until swelling subsides, but at least seven days	–
Poliomyelitis	YES	YES	Until certified well	Consult school doctor
Scarlet fever and other streptococcal infections of the nose and throat	YES / YES	YES (scarlet fever)	Until certified well	–
Tuberculosis	YES	YES	Consult school doctor	Consult school doctor
Gastro intestinal infections				
Dysentery	YES	YES	Until diarrhoea stops and as advised by school doctor	Consult school doctor

Disease	Notify		Cases – minimum period of exclusion	Contacts – necessary action
	School doctor	Medical Officer of Environmental Health		
Food poisoning (including salmonellosis)	YES	YES	Until diarrhoea stops and as advised by school doctor	Consult school doctor
Non specific gastroenteritis	YES	YES	Until diarrhoea stops and as advised by school doctor	Consult school doctor
Typhoid and para typhoid fever	YES	YES	Until bacteriologically clear	Consult school doctor
Skin diseases				
Impetigo or purulent eczema	YES	NO	Until healed	–
Plantar warts (verrucae)	YES	NO	Exclude from PE if painful	–
Ringworm of foot (athlete's foot)	YES	NO	Covered for PE	–
Ringworm of body (tinea)	YES	NO	Lesion should be covered	–

Disease	Notify		Cases – minimum period of exclusion	Contacts – necessary action
	School doctor	Medical Officer of Environmental Health		
Ringworm of scalp	YES	NO	Until certified clear	Consult school doctor
Scabies (caused by mites)	YES	NO	No exclusion once treatment has begun	Consult school doctor

Childhood Immunisation Programme, HN (85) 19, HN(FP) (85) 21 Health Notice, available from Health Publications Unit, No. 2 site, Manchester Road, Heywood, Lancs OL10 2PZ

Hygiene Precautions

In any situation where large numbers of people work in close proximity there is an ever present risk of outbreaks of certain infectious diseases. In special schools and those for younger children that risk is greater because of the increased likelihood of exposure to vomit, urine and excreta, and because such children may well have yet to develop satisfactory standards of personal hygiene. The possibility of outbreaks of disease can be minimised by the application of sensible hygiene precautions.

(a) A high standard of personal hygiene must be encouraged. Failure of pupils to wash their hands after using the toilet is the usual cause of outbreaks of bacillary dysentery and gastroenteritis, while similar lapses by kitchen staff can cause food poisoning cases. Soap, warm water and a means of drying hands must be available in sanitary accommodation and young pupils must be encouraged to use them.

(b) A small proportion of the population are carriers of infectious diseases. Many such carriers are unaware of their condition and the only sensible approach is to take adequate hygiene precautions in all cases.

(c) Staff should ensure that any cuts or broken skin are covered with waterproof or other suitable dressings while at work.

(d) Particular care must be taken when dealing with bleeding or other cases of spillage of body fluid:

  (i)   Disposable aprons and plastic gloves should be worn.

  (ii) Ordinary household bleach freshly diluted one to 10 parts water should be used for cleaning/disinfection purposes. (NB: Do not allow this solution to come into contact with skin or eyes. Flush with cold water if accidental contact occurs. Bleach may damage metal and fabrics if used at the wrong concentration.)

  (iii) Keep people away from the area until the spillage is dealt with.

  (iv) If the position of the spillage allows, carefully pour the diluted bleach over the area, cover with paper towels and leave for

30 minutes. If this is not an option, contaminated surfaces should be cleaned with liberal quantities of the above liquid.

(v)   Individual contaminated paper towels may be flushed down the toilet, but if a quantity has been used they, together with the gloves and apron, must be treated as infected waste.

(vi)   Infected waste, and that includes the disposable "nappy pads" used at some special schools, must not be placed in dustbins or paladins. If possible it should be incinerated on site. Where facilities for this are not available the waste must be placed in a yellow plastic sack and the local authority environmental health department approached to arrange for collection and disposal.

(vii)   On completion of work involving the cleaning up of body fluids hands should be thoroughly washed.

(e) Fears are sometimes expressed by first aiders about the possibility of their becoming infected with the Human Immunodeficiency Virus (HIV) when dealing with casualties. St John Ambulance Brigade and the British Red Cross have said that the precautions which have long been incorporated into their first aid training have proved to provide protection against blood borne infections. Their advice is:

(i)   First aiders should wash their hands before and after giving first aid.

(ii)   Any cuts or broken skin on their hands should be covered with waterproof plasters. If this is not possible disposable gloves should be worn.

(iii)   Any splashes of blood from another person on the skin, eyes or mouth should be washed off with copious amounts of water, or soap and water.

(iv)   If disposable gloves are worn the hands should be washed after first aid is given, firstly with the gloves on, and then again after the gloves are discarded.

(v)   There is no reason not to give mouth to mouth resuscitation for fear of being infected with HIV.

Smaller quantities of contaminated cotton wool, plasters, etc should be disposed of by flushing down the toilet. Heavyweight disposable gloves are inexpensive and there is little reason why they should not be provided for any first aider who is particularly concerned about possible infection, even if expert advice does not indicate that they are necessary.

(f) It is sensible to make arrangements to deal with vomit and urine spillages on school buses. Simple kits can be made up containing cat litter (to absorb fluids and to deodorise), a disposable tray and scraper, plastic bags, a small bottle of disinfectant, a cloth and disposable plastic gloves. (Care should be taken to ensure that the disinfectant used is not likely to damage metalwork or fabrics.)

Medicines and Pupils

When children are unwell the best place for them is at home with an adult. A sick child will not be able to cope with school activities, and if the illness is infectious there will be a serious risk of other children and staff becoming ill.

Occasionally, however, a doctor regards a child as fit to return to school provided a prescribed medicine is taken at midday. There are also children with long term illnesses who can only attend school if medication is either given during the school day or is available in an emergency. A small proportion of epilepsy sufferers require drugs at midday. All children with fibro-cystic disease must take medicine before all meals, and some children suffering with asthma need prescribed medication urgently in an attack.

Headteachers, while not wanting to deprive any child of the opportunity to attend school, are sometimes concerned about the legal implications of agreeing to dispense drugs in these circumstances. To do so is a straightforward discharge of their *in loco parentis* duty of care. It is, however, recommended that a written request, with details of the medicine involved, frequency of administration and dosage, be obtained from the parent.

It is first necessary to establish whether the LEA has any rules or conditions covering these circumstances. It is also wise to seek confirmation from the school doctor that the arrangements are both essential and satisfactory.

The parent must be responsible for providing the medicine in question in a suitable container clearly labelled with the child's name and directions for administration, and for replenishing supplies as necessary. The medicine must be kept under lock and key, with one designated member of staff being responsible for administering doses. The headteacher should keep a duplicate key in case of absences of the member of staff, etc. Drugs should be flushed down the toilet when no longer required.

When a pupil suffers from a disease such as epilepsy or asthma it is important that all members of staff who may come into contact with him or her are fully aware of the problem, of any limitations that need to be applied to the child's activities and what to do in an emergency. A note should be kept in the register to cover any possibility of this arrangement breaking down with supply teachers.

Analgesics

From time to time pupils suffer discomfort from toothaches, period pains, etc. It is not reasonable either to expect pupils to endure pain unnecessarily or to send them home in the middle of the day with the resulting loss of education. One LEA that decided to stop issuing analgesics quickly reversed its decision when it was found that some pupils were bringing bottles of tablets to school and dispensing them freely to their friends.

The provision of analgesics to pupils in a carefully controlled way is again no more than would be expected of a school discharging its *in loco parentis* duty of care.

Paracetamol, standard tablets for pupils of 12+ and in a children's form for younger pupils, is the only analgesic that should be administered in schools. Tablets should be given strictly according to the dosage specified on the container. They should be administered only by specifically authorised members of staff who should keep a simple record of all issues (eg name of child, time, dose given, brief reason). Analgesics must not be given to a pupil who is taking medication prescribed by a doctor. Paracetamol is a very dangerous drug in overdose. It must not be kept in first aid boxes or in any place accessible to pupils.

Further reading

Epilepsy—a Guide for Teachers
Epilepsy—the Package for Schools (Includes teachers' notes covering medical and practical aspects of the condition, pupils' materials, a poster covering first aid for persons with epilepsy and a book about a small boy with epilepsy.) Both the above publications are available from the British Epilepsy Association, 92 Tooley Street, London SE1.

Head Lice

Problems with head lice appear to have increased in frequency over recent years. While they are more of a nuisance than a health risk they can be a cause of much distress to parents, pupils and staff.

Adult lice move freely from host to host as head to head contact occurs. They lay their eggs close against the scalp glued to individual hairs. After hatching, the empty egg shell remains firmly attached to the hair, turns white and gradually becomes apparent as the hair grows. These shells are known as "nits". The difficulty of seeing the eggs at an early stage means that recognition of an infestation is unlikely until after hatching. It may be as long as three months after initial contact that itching occurs, although sometimes an allergic reaction to the faeces will occur earlier, producing a rash on the back of the neck and behind the ears, and hay fever type symptoms.

Lotions containing carbaryl or malathion kill the lice and eggs but do not affect the adhesion of the empty shells. These have to be drawn off by hand, an operation usually carried out with a fine-tooth comb.

Reinfestation readily occurs unless all cases are treated more or less simultaneously. Most parents accept the occasional outbreak as a normal hazard of childhood but become very distressed when repeated infestations are experienced. Some respond to such problems by regular precautionary use of insecticidal preparations, an unwise approach because of the risk of lice developing a resistance to the chemicals.

Health authorities throughout the country have policies for dealing with head lice infestation that vary slightly, but most agree that routine periodic head inspections are ineffective as a control measure. The responsibility for detection rests with parents and they should be advised to check their children's hair regularly. Parents should also be advised that the best precautionary measure is thorough brushing and combing of the hair last thing at night. Where infestation is suspected or confirmed advice and treatment should be sought from the school nurse or the local health centre. If an infestation remains unchecked, the Health Authority (contact the Senior Nursing Officer) will provide further assistance which may include full head inspections and arranging for visits to parents who need more specific advice and assistance.

Dermatitis

Dermatitis is the most frequent occupational health problem experienced in schools. Cleaners and kitchen staff are the main groups at risk but cases also occur in the art, CDT, home economics and science areas.

Irritant contact dermatitis (also known as irritant eczema) is a disease caused by direct action on the skin by chemicals, physical or biological agents. Symptoms include reddening of the skin, with possible peeling and puffiness, and blistering which may weep and produce crusting. Infection may set in, with pustule formation. If the chronic stage is reached the skin becomes thickened and the surface periodically flakes off. The effects are limited to the area that has been in contact with the substance in question and symptoms regress when contact with the substance ceases.

Allergic contact dermatitis (allergic eczema) is less common but is more serious in its effects and its implications. Initially the symptoms are similar to irritant contact dermatitis. After a few days' exposure, however, a complex reaction called sensitisation occurs. Subsequently, localised exposure to the substance produces a general reaction which may affect the entire skin surface of the sufferer. Approximately 20 per cent of the population are genetically predisposed to allergies and they are at risk of contracting this disease. Persons who suffer from asthma, hay fever or other allergies need to exercise particular care when handling substances known to be sensitising agents. Sensitisation may occur within a few days of the substance being first used but sometimes the condition is not triggered for a period of years. Reactions may occur at exposures considerably less than published occupational exposure limits which are intended to be levels that give reasonable freedom from health effects for the majority of workers. Once sensitisation has occurred complete avoidance of exposure to the causative agent will prevent further symptoms developing but this can have serious consequences if the agent is an essential element in the individual's work.

The Control of Substances Hazardous to Health Regulations 1988 requires employers to assess the health risks of substances used at work and includes the requirement that employees are informed of these risks. (See "Control of Substances Hazardous to Health Regulations".)

Substances used in schools that may produce irritant contact dermatitis include soaps, detergents, organic solvents, turpentine, soluble (cutting) oils, synthetic coolants, dyes, bleaches, various acids and alkalis, pesticides, white spirit, some plants and flowers, disinfectants and gum arabic.

Sensitising agents include epoxy, phenolic and acrylic resins, turpentine, fumes from resin fluxes, formaldehyde, fungicides, mercury, oil of clove, chromates and some photographic developers.

Prevention of dermatitis requires:

(a) where there is choice, selection of substances for use which have the least potential for causing harm
(b) careful observation of personal hygiene by staff using substances
(c) where necessary, the use of gloves and or barrier creams to help maintain the integrity of the skin
(d) the use of a proprietary hand cleaning product to remove heavy soiling, rather than pumice, hard soap and hard nail brushes
(e) the regular use of conditioning cream on skin that may have become defatted by exposure to substances, drying winds, or repeated or thorough washing following heavy soiling.

Further reading

Save Your Skin: Occupational Contact Dermatitis, MS(B)6, HSE 1987

Pregnancy

Pregnancy is a completely natural condition which should not unduly affect a woman's ability to continue with her work. Employers must recognise, however, that pregnancy does put extra strain on a working woman and all necessary steps must be taken to protect her and safeguard the unborn child. Staff working with children are exposed to infections which can be dangerous if contracted during pregnancy and the work of those who are normally expected to lift pupils may need to be modified if risk is to be avoided.

Rubella (German measles)

This is a mild infectious disease caused by a virus. Its symptoms are few and complications are rare. A mild fever, catarrhal symptoms, a rash of small, flat, pink spots mainly on the trunk and lasting only a day or two, and some swelling and tenderness of the glands on the back of the neck are typical indications. In perhaps 50 per cent of cases there are no apparent symptoms at all. Cases are contagious for about 16 days, eight days either side of the eruption of the rash. Immunity gained by an infection is long lasting.

If rubella is contracted during the first few months of pregnancy there is a serious risk to the foetus. Eye, ear and mental defects may result, and in perhaps 20 per cent of cases spontaneous abortion is caused.

All women who are likely to become pregnant can, and should, have a blood test to see whether they have a naturally acquired immunity. If the test proves negative their doctor can arrange immunisation. The best time for immunisation is in early adolescence and some education authorities have conducted vigorous campaigns to ensure that all girl pupils are protected.

In France, by ministerial decree, all teachers must be informed immediately of any case of rubella in a school and leave of absence must be given to any woman in the first four months of pregnancy who has a negative response to a seriological test. This is a reasonable approach given the risks involved.

The Burgundy Book provides that if an approved medical practitioner advises that a teacher in the early months of pregnancy should not attend her school because of the risk of exposure to rubella, and if the employer cannot provide reasonable alternative work at another school where there is no undue risk, the teacher will be granted leave with full pay.

Lifting and standing

Heavy lifting and long periods of continuous standing should be avoided by pregnant women. Lifting excessive weights may produce a sudden and abnormal increase in intra abdominal pressure with a risk of miscarriage or premature birth. In schools, work as diverse as lifting and carrying pupils, catering and cleaning may require some modification where a pregnant woman is concerned.

Visual display units (VDUs)

When VDUs were first introduced they were the subject of various stories in the media suggesting that they emitted harmful rays that caused miscarriages. With the passage of time and the widespread introduction of such equipment the Health and Safety Executive (HSE) in the United Kingdom, and the National Institution of Occupational Safety and Health in the USA, have carried out detailed and large scale studies of the possible health effects arising from the use of VDUs. Both studies showed that previous concerns had been unfounded. Unfortunately alarmist campaigns of the past have entered the folk memory. Women VDU users who are pregnant, or who are planning to become so, may suffer unnecessary stress and anxiety as a result. The HSE suggests that in such circumstances the woman should be given the opportunity to discuss her concerns with "someone adequately informed of current authorative scientific information and advice". In the first instance the employer should contact the local HSE Area Office (see HSE and Enforcement in Schools).

Rest Rooms

From 1 January 1996 pregnant women and nursing mothers at work must be provided with facilities to rest, and where necessary, to lie down. These facilities should be conveniently near sanitary accommodation. (Regulation 25, Workplace (Health, Safety and Welfare) Regulations 1992.)

Legal Aspects

The Sex Discrimination Act 1975 provides a waiver allowing discrimination where the unborn child might be at risk. The Congenital Disabilities (Civil Liability) Act 1976 allows a person to sue his or her mother's employers for any injurious effects resulting from the mother's employment during pregnancy. (The legislation also covers similar effects arising from the father's employment prior to conception.)

Proposals for an EC directive concerned with protecting the health and safety of pregnant workers, and workers who have recently given birth or who are breastfeeding are currently approaching the adoption stage. It is likely that regulations applying the requirements of the directive to the United Kingdom will be in place by the end of 1994.

Employers will be required to make an assessment of any risks to the health and safety of pregnant or breastfeeding workers arising from the workplace, using guidance to be provided. Pregnant workers, those likely to become pregnant and their safety representatives will be informed of the assessment results. If a risk is revealed the employer will be required either to adjust working conditions so that the risk is avoided or to move the worker to another job. if neither course is possible the worker will have to be given leave as necessary to protect her health and safety. The draft directive also contains provisions concerning maternity leave, time off for antenatal examinations and protection from dismissal because of pregnancy.

Further reading

Pregnancy and Work—Guidance for Women and Their Employers, MS(B)11, HSE 1989

Stress

Employers have a duty under the Health and Safety at Work, etc Act 1974 to take all reasonably practicable steps to protect the health, and that includes the mental health, of employees. Stress, or rather excessive stress, can produce emotional, physiological and behavioural reactions which can be damaging to health as well as reducing the employee's efficiency and effectiveness at work.

The human body is equipped to work at a wide range of levels in response to varying external influences. It may be likened to a petrol engine, ticking over quietly at normal levels of stress. When, however, excess stress is experienced the engine "revs up". This, again, is not an unhealthy condition in moderation but, like an engine, over-revving for too long produces premature wear and tear, which in turn causes a loss of efficiency. With reduced efficiency it is then necessary to over-rev just to produce an average performance, and so on until breakdown occurs.

There is still debate about whether excessive stress over a long period actually causes asthma, ulcers, heart disease, etc, or whether these are pre-existing conditions that are aggravated such that they manifest themselves. This is not really relevant because either way the end result is that the contribution made by the employee will have been reduced or lost, and his or her health and quality of life will have been harmed.

There are a number of factors which create excessive stress in schools, and victims may well react to several of them. It is often the case that when difficulties become superimposed on each other the total effect is greater than the sum of the effects. Ultimately, a comparatively minor additional stressor will prove to be the straw that breaks the camel's back. Typical factors are:

(a) work overload (too much work, unreasonable deadlines, insufficient time to allow a satisfying level of performance)
(b) undemanding work (lack of stimulus, few demands on creativity, too much routine)
(c) role conflicts (between home and work, between responsibility towards pupils and responsibility towards employer, between being a colleague and being an employee)
(d) lack of a sense of control (no say in how things are done, no consultation on matters about which the individual feels strongly, insecurity about reorganisations and closures)
(e) lack of self-confidence (feeling undervalued, fear of aggressive colleagues and pupils, feeling inadequate)
(f) lack of support and understanding (at home, from colleagues, parents and/or the headteacher)
(g) physical conditions (noise, too hot, too cold, queues to use toilets, crowded and uncomfortable staff rooms).

Excessive stress will produce changes in the behaviour of sufferers. Some may turn to alcohol or increase their use of tobacco, others may turn to patent medicines or overeat. Others become aggressive, violent and irrational, while some will become indifferent, uncaring and possibly indulge in absenteeism. Distress, anxiety and depression are common manifestations. The most telling indication of a stress problem is a change in normal behaviour and this should be considered as possibly indicating a need for assistance.

Events in life outside work can also be extremely stressful. Bereavements, divorces, family problems, etc experienced by staff require more than sympathy. Their short term impact on the total stress loading on the individuals concerned will be considerable and, where necessary, compensating adjustments should be made to their work.

Many education employers do little to try to minimise the factors that create excess stress even though any investment in this area is likely to be handsomely repaid. In the simplest terms, excess stress is caused by a poor "person/environment" match. The training of managers in person management, the introduction of systems for the early identification of problems and the provision of counselling, etc, recognition of the need to consider the effects on staff of change, and improving working conditions would go a long way towards eliminating this problem.

Further reading

Tackling Stress in Schools: a Practical Guide, Health Education Authority (an INSET training pack)
Cole M and Walker S, *Teaching and Stress*, Open University Press 1989
Gray H and Freeman A, *Teaching Without Stress*, Paul Chapman Publishing Ltd 1988
Managing Occupational Stress: A Guide for Managers in the Schools Sector, HSC 1990, HMSO
Teacher Stress: Where Do We Go From Here?, AMMA 1987
Stress In Teaching (conference report), AMMA 1988
Mental Distress at Work: First Aid Measures, IND(G) 129(L), HSE

Smoking in School

This is a subject capable of generating strong emotions and of causing serious damage to working relationships among staff unless dealt with sensitively. Teaching has the unenviable record of being the profession with the highest proportion of smokers in its ranks. Most schools ban smoking in the sight of pupils in the interests of not setting a bad example. These two factors combine together to produce a rush of smokers to the staff room at break times with, at the very least, an unpleasant effect on the environmental conditions there.

It seems unlikely that legislation will be introduced in the near future to control smoking at work. The Chairman of the Health and Safety Commission, when asked at a press conference in 1990 about the possibility of Government action, said "I am reluctant to get involved with regulations which we can't enforce". Various cases involving secondary smoking at work have been decided by industrial tribunals and it is sometimes asked why prosecutions have not been taken under the Health and Safety at Work, etc Act 1974. For such a case to succeed it would be necessary to prove beyond reasonable doubt that secondary smoking in the circumstances in question constituted a risk to health. The extent of current knowledge would make this very difficult. There is, however, no doubt whatever that smoking is a major cause of disease and premature death for smokers or that a woman who smokes during pregnancy puts her baby at risk. There is also no doubt that some persons who suffer from asthma and other respiratory disorders will suffer short term discomfort and distress if exposed to tobacco smoke laden air. What is less certain is the extent of the risk to non-smokers of serious harm arising from such exposure. Those medical experts who believe that secondary smoking can cause permanent harm say that only a very small proportion of non-smokers are likely to be so affected. Common sense suggests that people suffering harm in this way are likely to be those exposed to tobacco smoke for many hours per day over very many years.

Nonetheless, even if it were to be shown that no long term risk arises from exposure for only an hour a day it would be unlikely to stop the understandable objections of many non-smokers to having to share a staff room with smokers. The smell of tobacco smoke is unpleasant and it permeates furnishings and clothes. Rooms where people smoke quickly become dirty and require more frequent cleaning and decoration. There is also an increased fire risk in such areas.

Smoking appears to become a high profile issue sooner or later in most staff rooms and it is sensible for steps to be taken to minimise the likelihood of trouble before it arises. Where available space allows, a separate room should be provided for smokers. Failing this it may be possible to have a partition erected in the existing staff room, or to provide forced air extraction at one end of the room where smokers should be asked to gather. Total bans on smoking in staff rooms without some reasonable provision being made for those who wish, or need, to smoke are likely to cause problems. Consideration needs to be given to how such a ban would be enforced should a group of teachers decide to ignore it. Surreptitious smoking in areas not provided with ashtrays may well cause a fire risk, and ultimately staff may even resign and attempt to claim constructive dismissal. If this problem can be addressed before it reaches the last ditch stage it should be possible to achieve reasonable solutions without alienating sections of the staff.

Further reading

Passive Smoking at Work, IND(G)636, HSE 1988
Smoking Policies at Work, Health Education Authority (from HEA, Hamilton House, Mabledon Place, London WC1H 9TX)

Noise

Noise in schools may at times be a nuisance but only rarely is it likely to constitute a risk to anyone's hearing. Regulations designed to protect the hearing of people at work (the Noise at Work Regulations 1989) came into force on 1.1.90. They specify two levels of noise dose over a working day, and a level of instantaneous noise, which might present risks and detail the action to be taken when they are experienced.

Very high energy noise pulses of short duration may cause deafness. An action level of 200 pascals (140 db re 20 mpa) is specified for instantaneous noise peaks. This is a level of noise likely to be experienced when using explosive cartridge operated tools, on pistol ranges, etc.

Exposures to high average levels of noise over a period of years can also cause hearing loss. The action levels of 85 db(A) and 90 db(A) specified in the regulations mean either continuous noise at those levels over a full working day or fluctuating levels of noise, the average of which is equivalent to those levels. If, for example, someone is exposed to levels just above 85 db(A) for four hours and spends the rest of the day in comparative quiet the action level will not have been reached.

When it is considered that a domestic smoke alarm creates a noise of 85 db at a distance of one metre, and that at a 90 db(A) noise level it would be necessary to shout from a distance of 0.3 metre to communicate with 95 per cent intelligibility, it will be appreciated that few activities in schools present a risk in this respect.

Areas where problems may be experienced include:

(a) the use of tractors, grass cutting machines
(b) the use of chain saws
(c) the use of percussive drills
(d) the use of machines such as circular saws, continuously used for the majority of the day and on a regular basis.

Precision equipment is required to measure noise levels accurately. If a subjective assessment suggests that there might be a problem, expert help should be sought to determine the extent of any risk. LEA safety officers may have noise meters, as may environmental health officers from the local authority.

Where the noise dose exceeds 85 db(A) employers must provide ear protection if the employees ask for it. Where the 90 db(A) dose or the 200 pascal level are exceeded the employer must take all reasonably practicable steps to reduce the noise levels. If, despite this, those levels are still exceeded ear protection must be provided. There is a legal duty on the employer to see that it is used and on the employee to use it. Where such levels are experienced the area must be designated as an ear protection zone, marked with signs complying with the Safety Signs Regulations 1980, and employers must ensure that anyone entering the zone is wearing ear protection.

Where employees are exposed to daily average doses in excess of 85 db(A) the employer must provide the workers concerned with adequate information and instruction about the risks to hearing, how the risk can be minimised and what their responsibilities are under the regulations.

Potentially dangerous sound levels can be produced by the high powered equipment used at discos and concerts in schools. While such exposures are likely to be only occasional it is sensible to minimise any possible risk by keeping people away from a two or three metre area in front of loudspeakers and to keep the level down to about 90 db(A), using the subjective assessment described above.

Regulation 12 modifies the duty placed on suppliers by s.6(1) of the Health and Safety at Work, etc Act 1974. Machinery manufacturers and suppliers are now required to provide noise data with any machine likely to cause exposures above 85 db(A) or the 200 pascals level.

Further reading

Humphrey, J and Farmer, D *Too Loud*, Croner 1990
Noise at Work—Advice for Employees, IND(G) 99(L), HSE
Training and Competence Standards for Users of Chainsaws, Guidance Note GS48, HSE, HMSO

Cleaning in Pottery Areas

Clay contains silica, a material which if inhaled will cause damage which reduces the efficiency of the lungs. In its normal damp state there is no risk of respirable dust being released. If, however, clay is allowed to dry out and is then machined or scarified a potentially dangerous situation is created. Cleaning staff are particularly at risk if sweeping of floors contaminated with dry clay is permitted.

A combination of measures are necessary to eliminate any risk. Pottery room floors should be cleaned either by a wet washing method or, if the construction of the floor does not permit this, by use of a vacuum cleaner fitted with a special filter capable of stopping particles down to one micron in size. (NB: nuisance dust masks offer no protection against particles of a size that will be harmful.) Shelves should only be cleaned with a damp cloth. Users of such areas should minimise any risk by cleaning up spills of slip before it dries out. Any cloths used for this purpose must be kept damp. Floors in pottery rooms should be cleaned daily, while kiln rooms and shelving in pottery rooms should be cleaned at least once per half term.

Further reading

Silica Dust and You, MS(A)15, HSE

Health & Safety (Display Screen Equipment) Regulations 1992

These regulations are intended to improve the working practices, equipment and environment of employees who use "display screen equipment" for a significant proportion of their working day and are at risk of suffering musculoskeletal or visual fatigue, and mental stress problems as a result.

Whether the specific requirements of these regulations or the more general requirements of the Management of Health and Safety at Work Regulations 1992 apply to a worker depends on the specified definitions of "user" and "display screen equipment". A "user" is an employee who "habitually uses" display screen equipment as a significant part of his or her work. "Display screen equipment" covers cathode ray tube and liquid crystal displays whose main use is to show text and/or graphics, and systems such as microfiche. (Window typewriters, lap top computers and calculators are among specific exclusions.) Numerous examples are given in the guidance note, from which it is certain that a school secretary, using a display screen type word processor typically for two or more hours per day is a "user". A librarian who either uses "display screen equipment" intensively on most days, or more intermittently "but still forming at least half of his or her total working time" will also be a "user". However a teacher employing such equipment for preparing handouts would only be considered so if periods of use were frequent, of long duration and intensive.

Where there is a possibility that an employee meets the definition of "user" the employer must arrange for an assessment of risks arising from the workstation in question, reduce risks thus exposed so far as is reasonably practicable, and have the assessment reviewed when necessary. Assessments should be carried out by a competent person (see "Consultants") who should make a written record of the findings, and should involve the "user" and the user's safety representative in the assessing process.

Regulation 3 specifies that any workstation for a "user" first put into service after 1 January 1993 meets requirements (in respect of the equipment, the desk, the chair, working space, lighting, etc, noise, temperature, humidity, and the software) spelled out in the schedule to the regulations. Existing workstations must be improved as necessary to meet these requirements by the end of 1996. (If new display screen equipment is introduced during the transitional period, the whole workstation must be brought into compliance immediately. If any other component, such as a chair, is changed it must comply at once but the rest of the workstation need not comply until December 1996.)

Employers are required by Regulation 4 to ensure that the work of users is planned so that tasks involving display screen equipment is periodically interrupted by spells of non-display screen work or formal breaks, to prevent fatigue and to vary visual and mental demands.

Where a person is a user on 1 January 1993, or is to become a user, he or she can request an eye and eyesight test, which must be arranged as soon as is practicable and at the employer's expense. Regulation 5 also requires that further such tests are to be made available at regular intervals (as recommended by the optometrist), and if and when users subsequently experience eyestrain or focusing difficulties which might be due to their work. The employer must meet the cost of any special corrective appliances needed where ordinary reading/distance type appliances are not satisfactory for the work in question. ("Ordinary" type appliances are at the user's own expense.) Where users are prescribed a special pair of spectacles exclusively for display screen work the employer's liability for the cost is limited to payment for a basic appliance, of a type and quality adequate for its function.

Regulation 6 requires employers to provide users, and those who are to become users, with training in the health and safety implications of their workstations. Further such training must be provided when there is any significant change to the workstation.

Employers must also provide (Regulation 7) information to users about the health and safety aspects of their workstations, the assessments described above, and steps taken to comply with Regulations 3, 4 and 6.

The Health and Safety Executive has published very detailed guidance on these regulations in *Display Screen Equipment Work*.

It must be emphasised that working with display screen equipment does not cause eye defects or make worse existing defects. However an uncorrected defect, of which the user may previously have been unaware, is likely to cause quite severe, if temporary, problems when such visually demanding work is undertaken.

While this legislation does not apply to pupils, and the extent of their use of display screen equipment, even in secondary schools, would not constitute a risk to their health or safety, many of them will go on to use such equipment in later life. A strong case can be made for pupils to be taught about correct posture and appropriate keying techniques so that bad habits are not passed from school to the workplace.

Further reading

Display Screen Equipment Work, HMSO 1992
Working with VDUs, IND(G) 36L, HSE 1992

Chapter 13
Fire

Introduction

There is a need for constant vigilance by all staff in schools to ensure that life and property are not endangered by fire. While to date the record of schools has been good so far as personal injury is concerned the same cannot be said in respect of premises. Tens of millions of pounds worth of damage to schools occurs each year and a high proportion of these fires are due to arson. The waste, loss of facilities and the risks to life so caused do not need spelling out.

Regulation 7, Management of Health and Safety at Work Regulations 1992, requires schools to set up and put into effect appropriate arrangements for the evacuation of premises in emergencies such as fire. This legislation also requires that employees, contractors' employees, temporary workers and agency workers working on the premises are given information, in a comprehensible form, about those arrangements.

The Fire Precautions Act 1971 allowed for the subsequent designation of types of premises which would require a fire certificate from the fire authority. Schools have not yet been so designated and a certificate is not required at the time of writing.

The local fire authority is responsible for enforcement of most aspects of legislation relating to fire but where fires occur at a place of work the Health and Safety Executive (HSE) may be involved. The HSE must be informed where a fire involving materials used at work, their by products or finished products results in the suspension of work in the area for more than 24 hours. (Reporting of Injuries, Diseases and Dangerous Occurrences Regulations 1985. See "Accidents".)

Fire prevention officers of the local fire brigade will usually be found to be most helpful in providing specific advice relating to evacuation of premises, types and numbers of extinguishers that are required, fire alarms, access for fire engines, etc. In inner London, for example, they agreed to attend one fire drill per school each year.

Every school should have detailed, written regulations covering all aspects of emergency evacuations. The headteacher, in consultation with colleagues, the school safety committee and the fire brigade should have drawn up and submitted to the governors for approval a document covering the following points:

(a) the steps to be taken by anyone discovering a fire and after the alarm has been given
(b) how the fire brigade is to be summoned
(c) the evacuation procedure, including the arrangements for areas such as kitchens, laboratories, swimming pools, etc
(d) any special circumstances relating to the premises which need to be considered (eg use of lifts)
(e) the evacuation of people with disabilities.

Once approved by the governors, the regulations should become part of the school's statement of health and safety arrangements. They must be explained to, and understood by, all staff, both teaching and non-teaching, and it is sensible to keep a written record to prove that this procedure has been carried out. Headteachers should regularly review and revise the regulations in the light of experience, taking into account reorganisations of the school, temporary or permanent changes of use of areas, etc.

Evacuation of Premises

There are two basic methods of providing for the efficient evacuation of numbers of people from a building in an emergency. Where the people concerned are the same over long periods of time, and it is known exactly who is on the premises, the fire drill/roll call system can be employed. Where, however, premises are used in the evenings or at weekends by groups of people who may not be familiar with the layout of the school or the drill procedures the signed route system must be employed.

The "signed route" system requires that at any location within corridors, on stairways, and in areas such as halls that have more than one exit, it is possible to see a sign that indicates the appropriate evacuation route from that point. This system requires that a physical check of the premises is made to confirm they have been fully evacuated. A similar check will be necessary when using the fire drill method at those times during the day, such as lunchtime, when it may well not be possible to establish that total evacuation has been achieved by a roll call. In both cases the person in charge must advise the fire brigade immediately on their arrival whether there are any persons unaccounted for.

Fire Alarms

Every school must have a suitable method of warning everyone on the premises that an evacuation is to take place. The alarm may be given by electrical bells, electronic signals via loudspeakers, sirens, or even by hand bells, but whatever the method it is essential that the signals are audible in each and every location where a person might be on the premises. This includes sanitary accommodation, boiler houses and store-rooms, and rest rooms where, perhaps, someone feeling unwell might be asleep.

Electrical and electronic systems should be tested each day before school hours by the caretaker, and any defects reported to the headteacher on arrival. Additionally, there should be a monthly check at a published time during working hours to enable members of staff to ensure audibility throughout the school.

False alarms are a problem in some schools and it has been known for headteachers to switch off alarms rather than endure continual disruption. A wiser course is to arrange for a modification to the system so that a short delay is introduced to allow the correctness of the alarm call to be established before the evacuation signal is sounded. One headteacher quickly eliminated false alarms by starting a stopwatch whenever he left his desk, stopping it on his return and adding the elapsed time onto the end of the school day!

School safety committees can make a valuable contribution to fire safety by monitoring the effectiveness of the school's arrangements and fire matters should be a fixed agenda item for their meetings.

Fire Drills

Where LEAs specify the number of drills that are to be carried out this must be complied with. Where such instructions are not given, six practice evacuations per year may be considered to be a reasonable number. The first drill should be held as soon as possible after the start of the academic year, two others in that term, two in the spring term and one in the summer term. Except for the first drill in the year, all drills should be held without warning and staff and pupils should not know that it is a drill until roll calls are completed.

If a false alarm occurs, the building should be fully evacuated before reoccupation. It may be decided to allow such an evacuation to proceed to a roll call and to count it as one of the quota for the term.

For each fire drill a notional location for the fire should be determined and the "danger" area closed to people leaving the building. This will train staff and pupils to use alternative routes as circumstances dictate.

On reaching the assembly area teachers must quickly establish that all pupils are accounted for and notify the headteacher of any that are missing.

Once the premises have been evacuated no one should be allowed to re-enter without the permission of the senior member of staff present. Where the police or fire brigade are present the senior member of staff must seek such permission from the officer in charge.

Drills through the year should be held at different times, so that problems that arise during assemblies and at break times can be identified and countered as necessary.

Where there is a kitchen on the premises the catering staff must be fully involved in the arrangements for emergency evacuation. It would not, however, be reasonable to allow a meal to be ruined because of a drill. The headteacher should consult the head of kitchen about such possibilities and where necessary arrange that only a representative of the kitchen staff takes part in the practice. At least twice per year drills should be held at times that permit all kitchen staff to join in.

The headteacher should keep a record of all drills held, with details of the time taken to vacate the premises and any difficulties experienced. This information should be included in a report to the next ordinary governors' meeting.

Means of escape

A means of escape is a continuous route along which persons can travel by their own efforts from any place that they may find themselves within a building to the safety of the open air at ground level. In schools the usual requirement is that the maximum distance between any point in the building and safety does not exceed 50 metres. In a multi-storey building "safety" will mean a protected staircase. Protected staircases are enclosed structures designed to have a significantly greater fire resistance than the rest of the building and to be smoke proof. The minimum width of escape routes are determined according to the maximum number of persons who may use the route in an emergency. Escape routes must be constructed so as to allow occupants time to use them. Thus, doors opening onto an escape route have to be of suitable fire resistance, the surfaces of walls must not support the spread of fire and cross corridor doors have to be provided at appropriate places to stop the spread of smoke.

An alternative means of escape is only required from a room if it is an assembly room likely to have more than 60 people present, if it is a laboratory or other high fire risk room, if a single door would be in a hazardous position, if any part of the room is more than 12 metres in a straight line to the door, or if the room opens into another room which is a high fire risk area. It can be seen that the rules are complicated. Determination of what is satisfactory also depends on other factors which require technical expertise and judgement, and specialist advice should be sought where any doubt exists. It is, however, obvious that schools need to take care to avoid compromising the means of escape features designed into the building. The width of escape routes must not be reduced by the introduction of cupboards or other furniture. If pupils' work is fixed to corridor walls gaps of 0.5 metre should be left every two metres to prevent the spread of flame. Smoke stop doors must be maintained in good condition and kept closed except when classes are actually passing through them. Expert advice should be obtained before areas are altered by the erection of partitions, etc which may alter travel distances and/or introduce materials which do not meet fire resistance requirements. Lastly, but certainly not least, fire exit doors must be unlocked while the premises are occupied

There is often a conflict between the needs of security and means of escape. Some large schools have far too many entrances to allow for proper control and there may be good reasons to consider securing those which are not required for means of escape. Where intruders are a problem, special locks and fittings are available for fire exits which permit ready egress whilst preventing unwanted entry. The advice of the fire brigade should be sought before any such measures are put into effect (see "Violence and Security").

Escape lighting

Confusion exists between escape and emergency lighting. Emergency lighting is provided in work places (eg operating theatres, broadcasting studios) where it is necessary to continue work despite a power failure. Escape lighting simply provides sufficient illumination to allow persons to evacuate premises safely in the event of a power failure, a situation which may well arise in a fire. Any building which is used outside daylight hours should have an effective means of allowing safe evacuation in such circumstances. The level of light necessary is only dim moonlight and various methods can be used to provide this. Ideally trickle charged battery powered lights which switch on automatically if the power fails are permanently fixed on all escape routes. Some fire authorities may agree to the use of photoluminescent tapes and discs which emit a remarkable amount of light for an hour or so after being energised by light. These are automatic in effect, require no maintenance and are comparatively inexpensive to install. Failing all else or as a temporary expedient, a sufficient number of torches or lanterns to facilitate evacuation will need to be available to the persons in charge of evening activities.

Signs and notices

To comply with the Safety Signs Regulations 1980 all signs indicating a safe condition must be green with white lettering. This applies to all fire exit and means of escape directional signs. Signs indicating the location of fire alarms, hose reels, etc are coloured red with white lettering.

Where fire exit and directional signs should be located is described above under "Evacuation of Premises". For other fire signs it is important to avoid an over-enthusiastic approach which may reduce the impact of necessary signs, waste money and impinge on the general environment. There is no point, for example, in putting a sign that says "fire bucket" over a red painted bucket filled with sand. It is, however, necessary to indicate where a fire alarm call point may be found if this is not reasonably apparent. Common sense should prevail in cases of doubt.

Self-adhesive vinyl signs are less expensive than rigid metal or PVC types but they may prove to be a false economy if they can be reached by pupils. Photoluminescent signs are available and their extra cost is justifiable because they are clearly visible in those dark conditions which may be experienced when their help is needed most.

Notices giving details of fire regulations, fire alarm systems and assembly points are usually displayed in classrooms, offices and corridors. Such notices should be as brief as possible, giving only essential information and should be highly legible. Experience suggests that the only time they are likely to be read by most people is when an alarm signal is heard and they are unsure what to do.

Where school premises are used by members of the public the person in charge should be instructed to bring the arrangements for emergency evacuations to their attention at an early stage in the proceedings.

Fire fighting equipment

Equipment appropriate for the type of fire risk in each area should be provided for use in emergency situations.

Staff should be instructed never to put themselves at risk in attempting to fight a fire.

Fire fighting equipment requires regular maintenance and inspection. School caretakers should keep a log of all equipment, etc and record details of annual maintenance checks. It is usual practice for a manila label to be tied to each extinguisher, to be signed and dated by the person carrying out the check.

The fire brigade will provide specific advice on the type and level of extinguisher provision required.

Cases have occurred where children have died as a result of using BCF extinguishers in solvent abuse experiments. This type of extinguisher should not be specified for any area or in vehicles to which pupils have access.

People with disabilities

Over recent years there has been a movement towards the increased use of school premises by people with physical disabilities for both education and employment purposes. While such initiatives are to be welcomed, careful consideration must be given to the means of ensuring their reasonable safety, especially where emergency evacuations are concerned.

Under the Chronically Sick and Disabled Persons Act 1970 all subsequently built school buildings were required to make provision for the ready access and other needs of disabled persons. Many older buildings, however, present serious difficulties in these respects and satisfactory solutions need to be worked out in advance of any commitments being made to disabled people.

The advice of the fire brigade should be obtained when considering the various possibilities. Where single storey buildings are concerned, or where a non-ambulant person will only have access to the ground floor, the provision of adequate ramps on all means of escape routes may be all that is needed. In some multi-storey buildings a special evacuation, or "fireman's", lift is or can be provided. Unlike most lifts these are specially designed to allow for their use in fire situations without risk. Depending on the layout of the building, the fire brigade might agree to the movement of a disabled person to a place of comparative safety on an upper floor, pending rescue by themselves on arrival. A place of comparative safety might be a lobby within a protected staircase area or, in a building with two or more separate wings, in an unaffected part of the premises.

For multi-storey buildings that do not have a place of comparative safety, evacuation chairs might be considered. These are wheelchairs fitted with rubber belts that can safely be taken down a staircase by one person. They are designed so that the heavier the person in the chair the greater the braking effect. They can only be used for descending stairs and are of value only where a lift is available to give normal access to upper floors. If this method is adopted it is essential that there is always someone available in the immediate vicinity of the disabled person to assist in an emergency. When a general evacuation is taking place it will be necessary for the person wheeling the chair to wait until the majority of people have passed down the stairs before descending if undue congestion is to be avoided.

Where disabled children are concerned carrying down stairs might be considered as an answer. Again, this requires precise and sure management arrangements so that volunteers are readily and always available.

While arranging for the safe evacuation of non-ambulant persons is perhaps the greatest challenge, the safety of people with other disabilities must also be considered. The deaf may not be able to hear alarm signals, partially sighted or blind people may sometimes have to use exit routes with which they are not familiar, and people with special learning difficulties may require guidance. A system of escorts should be established, with substitutes to cover absences due to leave or sickness, etc.

Before finalising special arrangements for disabled people it is important that the agreement of the fire brigade be obtained, and that evacuation by whatever method is agreed is realistically rehearsed.

(Regulations in response to an EC directive are currently in preparation. To be made under the Fire Precautions Act 1971, they are likely to require that an assessment is made of all workplaces by experts in fire safety matters. It is understood that delays have occurred because of difficulties in determining issues such as who will be responsible for enforcement of the new legislation.)

Further reading

Fire and the Design of Schools, DES, 5th edn., HMSO 1975
A Guide to Fire Safety in Schools, Scottish Education Department, HMSO 1979
Croner's Fire Record Keeping Book, Croner 1990

Chapter 14
Welfare Provision

First Aid

First aid is a statutory welfare provision. The Health and Safety at Work, etc Act 1974 (HASAWA) provides for the "health, safety and welfare" of employees but only the "health and safety" of non-employees at a place of work (ie pupils). The Health and Safety (First Aid) Regulations 1981 were made under the HASAWA and it was therefore not technically possible for the question of provision for pupils to be addressed in this legislation.

A revised Approved Code of Practice and Guidance which included a number of changes in the interpretation of the Regulations was published in 1990. The original threshold for the provision of a trained first aider at a school (150 employees at work) has been amended to 50 employees (ie one first aider if there are more than 50 employees at work, two if there are more than 100, and so on). Other changes have been made in training requirements and the contents of first aid boxes.

While there remains no requirement under the regulations to take pupils into account, schools have, of course, a moral and a civil law duty to make reasonable provision for them.

First aiders

It is difficult for many headteachers to determine, in the absence of any laid down scale, what is a reasonable minimum level of provision for their school. In 1982 the Inner London Education Authority (ILEA) set up a scheme with the following ratios:

	Minimum
No. of persons regularly on site	*no. of first aiders*
Up to –349	1
350–699	2
700–999	3
1000–1499	4
1500–1999	5

After approximately 10,000 school/years' experience there was no evidence that such a level of provision was inadequate. It must, however, be said that the ILEA was operating in an inner city area with excellent National Health Service (NHS) facilities. For those of its establishments located more than seven miles away from an NHS casualty department, and in schools for ESN(S), physically handicapped, delicate and visually handicapped pupils, the specified level was increased to at least two trained first aiders, irrespective of numbers of persons on site.

The Health and Safety Executive has said that it is happy with arrangements that combine cover for statutory and non-statutory areas provided that there is no dilution of the statutory provision for employees.

To meet a statutory requirement, first aiders have to be trained to a standard approved by the Health and Safety Executive. In practice this means an initial four day course run by one of the approved training organisations (eg British Red Cross, St John Ambulance), with a two day refresher course every three years. From 1990 a new section has been included in the training syllabus about protection against blood borne viral infections such as hepatitis B and HIV.

In seeking volunteers to be trained, headteachers should bear in mind that calm, cautious and responsible individuals able to cope with an intensive course of study will make the best first aiders. It is sensible to endeavour to spread first aid cover across the main areas of activity of the school. It is also preferable to avoid selecting members of staff with a heavy teaching commitment for this purpose. If it proves difficult to find volunteers consideration should be given to writing the task into the job description of the next non-teaching staff member recruited.

Concern is sometimes expressed about the legal position of first aiders if they should cause injury to a casualty. An employer is vicariously liable for the negligent actions of employees who are acting within the scope of their employment. Cover against any award of damages in such circumstances is provided by the employer's liability insurance. Staff can be reassured in this respect, whether they are trained first aiders or not, provided that they endeavour to act in the best interests of the employer. (See "Vicarious Liability" and "Employers Liability (Compulsory Insurance) Act 1969").

First aid boxes

The regulations require that first aid materials are readily available to all employees. Due regard must be paid to meeting this requirement in respect of persons such as cleaners who work on the premises outside normal hours. The permitted contents of first aid boxes are restricted to those items that can be used by an untrained person to treat themselves and others without risk of exacerbating injuries. "Statutory" first aid boxes may contain *only* the following items:

(a) a printed card listing the contents and a leaflet giving general guidance on first aid
(b) individually wrapped sterile dressings
(c) sterile eye pads with attachment
(d) triangular bandages (sterile or, if not, with suitable sterile coverings for serious wounds)
(e) safety pins
(f) selection of medium, large and extra large sterile unmedicated dressings
(g) where mains tap water is not immediately available at least 900 ml of sterile water, or sterile normal saline solution, should be provided.

First aid boxes should be constructed so as to ensure that the contents are kept clean and dry, and labelled with a white cross on a green background so as to be easily identifiable. Disposable plastic gloves (see "Hygiene") should be stored near the first aid boxes.

First aid kits must be available to groups taking part in outside activities. The guidance states that "travelling first aid kits" should contain at least a card giving general advice on first aid, six individually wrapped sterile adhesive dressings, one large sterile unmedicated dressing, two triangular bandages, two safety pins, and individually wrapped moist cleaning wipes. (The wipes should not be impregnated with alcohol.)

When the regulations were first published there was concern that the limitations of first aid materials would make it difficult to care properly for pupils in the *in loco parentis* role, and especially in boarding schools. After much debate the DES issued a bulletin authorising the provision of additional items to trained first aiders, subject to the approval of the LEA medical officer/school doctor, and to such items not being kept in the statutory first aid boxes. A typical list of additional items would be:

(a) crêpe bandages
(b) roller bandages
(c) cotton wool
(d) forceps or tweezers
(e) scissors
(f) kidney dish
(g) centrimide antiseptic cream (eg Savlon)
(h) centrimide antiseptic suitably diluted for use
(i) tie on labels
(j) 14″ diameter plastic bowl
(k) notebook and pencil.

Responsibility for maintaining the contents of first aid boxes is usually delegated to the school's first aiders.

Appointed persons

The regulations require that where a first aider is not appointed or is absent there must be an "appointed person" to act in his or her stead. Where there is a statutory requirement for a first aider (ie at least 50 employees at work) employers cannot rely on an appointed person to cover for foreseeable absences such as leave.

In larger schools this may mean that if there is just one trained first aider that individual cannot be permitted to take annual leave during term time. During holiday periods and for activities at weekends, in the evenings, etc when there are not 50 employees on site the legal requirement can be met by an appointed person. This role is usually carried out by the caretaker outside normal school hours.

The Approved Code of Practice says that the appointed person should "ideally" be trained in emergency first aid. His or her main task is to take charge of the situation in the event of serious injury or illness, to ensure that an ambulance is summoned and that a responsible person is sent to open any gates and to direct the ambulance crew to the casualty. Such a person should direct pupils away from the area, and obtain from the crew details of where the casualty is being taken, and subsequently ensure that parents are notified and that the appropriate accident reporting procedures are put in train.

Ambulances

While it is not essential that a responsible adult accompanies a child who is taken from school by ambulance it is highly desirable that this be arranged if at all possible. Failing this, a brief note giving details of the accident/illness, together with the child's name and address, should be given to the ambulance crew and parents informed as soon as practicable. *On no account should provision of urgently needed medical treatment be delayed pending the arrival at school of parents, etc.*

Schools should liaise with the local ambulance service to minimise delays in emergency situations.

First aid room

While there is not a statutory requirement for a first aid room in a school it may be convenient to use an existing medical examination room for this purpose. The Approved Code of Practice spells out the facilities that have to be provided where there is a legal requirement and schools may choose to adopt some or all of these.

Notices

Details of arrangements for first aid and for dealing with serious injury/ illness, should be spelled out in the school statement and brought to the attention of all staff. In every school there must be at least one notice published in a conspicuous place giving details of who the first aider is and where he or she can be located. In larger schools such notices should be posted in each area or department. Notices, coloured green and white and providing spaces for names, etc, are available commercially.

Further reading

First Aid in Educational Establishments, HMSO 1985
First Aid at Work: General First Aid Guidance for First Aid Boxes, HMSO
First Aid at Work, COP 42, HSC 1990, HMSO

Lighting

Lighting tends only to be noticed when it is unsatisfactory. Adequate, well designed and maintained lighting makes an important contribution to work efficiency, to health and safety and to the creation of a satisfactory visual environment.

The Education (School Premises) Regulations 1981 gives statutory weight to the main recommendations on lighting given in the DES Design Note 17 *Guidelines for Environmental Design and Fuel Conservation in Educational Buildings*. Schools should be lit by daylight whenever and wherever possible. Artificial light will be provided to accommodate variations in daylight conditions. Two main types of artificial lighting are used in schools. Incandescent lamps are, however, gradually being superseded by fluorescent fittings which are less wasteful of electricity, require less frequent attention and provide a light that approximates more closely to daylight. Problems are sometimes experienced when this changeover is made. Complaints of headaches and general malaise will occur unless the new installation has been correctly designed. More often than not the problem is too much light. (In one classroom it was found to be necessary to remove half the newly installed fluorescent tubes to achieve a satisfactory level of lighting. Electricians are rarely also lighting design engineers.) Where the ceiling of a room is low and fittings are in the line of vision glare will be a problem, as it may if light reflects from shiny work surfaces.

Design Note 17 specifies a minimum illuminance of 150 lux at any point on the work surface whatever the light source, not less than 300 lux where fluorescent lamps are used and not less than 350 lux where lighting is achieved by a mixture of artificial and daylight. The Chartered Institution of Building Services, in its *Code for Interior Lighting 1984*, recommends levels of 300 lux in halls, classrooms, libraries, gymnasia and workshops, and 500 lux in art rooms, needlerooms (with supplementary local lighting) and laboratories.

Fluorescent lighting could cause a problem when used in workplaces where there is machinery with exposed moving parts. The light is actually flickering at a frequency too great for the eye to see. If it illuminates a moving object and the frequency of rotation of the object matches, or is a multiple, or sub multiple, of the frequency of the light the stroboscopic effect is seen. This creates the illusion that the moving part is stationary or moving very slowly, and this could be dangerous. In such areas alternate light fittings should be wired on different supply phases, or high frequency fittings should be used.

It is not generally appreciated that the light output from fluorescent tubes will decline by as much as 10 per cent over 2500 hours of usage. Further reductions in illumination are caused by dirt on walls, the ceiling, and the light fitting—perhaps 15 per cent after three years in a room of average cleanliness with semi-direct lighting. It can be seen that from an economic as well as a health and safety viewpoint it is important that fittings are cleaned regularly (typically annually in August) and that tubes are replaced periodically as a batch rather than waiting for them to stop working. (Manufacturers will advise on the point in a tube's life when it is most economic for it to be replaced.)

A problem arose in some schools where lighting was being changed from incandescent to fluorescent. It was alleged that because fluorescent lights emit ultra violet light they would put the pupils at risk of developing skin cancer. Measurements made showed that there was no emission when diffusers were fitted. When these were removed it was found that the total dose over a year would be equivalent to that which would be experienced in one hour out of doors on a sunny day. (See also Regulation 8, Workplace (Health, Safety and Welfare) Regulations 1992, and Regulation 21, Provision and Use of Work Equipment, 1992.)

Further reading

Guidelines for Environmental Design and Fuel Conservation in Educational Buildings, Design Note 17, DES 1981
Code of Interior Lighting, Chartered Institution of Building Services 1984
Lighting at Work, HMSO, 1987

Temperatures

The Education (School Premises) Regulations 1981 (SI 909) give statutory weight to recommendations in respect of the temperatures that should be maintained in schools which had been previously published in DES Design Note 17. The specified temperatures are intended to reflect typical levels of activity and the amount of clothing likely to be worn. The temperatures are:

(a) in areas where there will be an average level of activity and an average level of clothing (eg classrooms, all-purpose halls in primary schools) 18°C

(b) in areas where persons are lightly clad and inactive (eg medical rooms, changing rooms) 21°C

(c) in areas where occupants are lightly clad but where activity is vigorous (eg gymnasia) 14°C

(NB: where gymnasia are used for examinations during the heating season the heating should be capable of adjustment to 18°C or arrangements made to provide supplementary heating.)

(d) the temperature of circulation spaces, corridors, etc should be within 3°C of the area that they serve

(e) in dormitories 15°C

(f) in areas where occupants have a lower than usual rate of activity because of physical disability 21°C.

These levels are higher than those required in adult workplaces under other legislation because children, with lower body weights, are less able to withstand cold than are adults.

From 1 January 1996 (immediately in new premises) the Workplace (Health, Safety and Welfare) Regulations 1992 (W(HSW)R) will require that reasonable temperatures are maintained and that thermometers are provided to allow staff to check that this is done. "Reasonable temperatures" in areas used by adults for sedentary work will be at least 16°C.

Heating systems are designed to provide a given temperature lift above a usual minimum winter temperature, normally –1°C. It would not be reasonable to design systems to cope with conditions which may occur, say, once in 50 years, and in unusually cold periods it may not be possible to achieve the specified levels. At such times it may be necessary to forgo the economies gained by time switches and to leave the heating on for 24 hours a day, six days per week and/or to provide supplementary heating.

Subjective assessments of the adequacy of heating are often inaccurate. Where minor problems are suspected the temperature in the area should be measured hourly and the figures recorded, over a period of a few days. If the record obtained confirms any shortcomings it will also be of assistance to the heating engineer.

Supplementary/emergency heating

From a safety and convenience viewpoint the preferred type of heater for these purposes is the electrical convector heater. The only limiting factor on the use of such appliances is the ability of the electrical circuits in the school to provide sufficient power.

Paraffin or Calor gas heaters are possible alternatives where electrical convector heaters cannot be employed. Both types are potentially hazardous and should only be used with strict precautions in force. Paraffin heaters must be screwed down to the floor and be fitted with a wire guard to prevent pupils touching them. The fuel must be kept outside the building in a secure store and tanks must not be refilled inside the building. Considerable damage can be caused by a badly adjusted flame filling an area with carbon-rich smoke and close supervision is necessary. The use of Calor gas heaters in schools has been the subject of advice from the Health and Safety Executive (*Temporary Use of Liquefied Petroleum Gas Heaters in Schools*, HSE 1986). Both paraffin and Calor gas heaters can only be safely operated in areas which are adequately ventilated.

Regulation 7, W(HSW)R, requires that after 1 January 1996 (in most schools) the method of heating will be such as "to avoid the escape into the workplace of injurious or offensive fumes, gas or vapour", a standard obviously deserving immediate application.

Thermal gain

DES Design Note 17, referred to above, also states that schools should be designed so as to avoid temperatures within the building exceeding 27°C on more than 10 days in any year. Thermal gain problems can be severe, particularly in the glass and concrete structures erected in the 1960s, and rectification can be difficult and extremely expensive. Although temperatures in classrooms reaching 30°C may not cause anything more than short term and minor ill health effects it will certainly have a serious effect on the education process.

In some schools thermal gain problems are experienced throughout the year whenever the sun shines. A number of solutions are available. External blinds are effective but expensive to maintain. Internal blinds will cure glare problems but will do little to reduce heat build-up. Special glass, and film that is applied to existing glass, can also be effective but some types give the outside world a depressing grey cast. *In extremis* a cheap and effective but short term expedient is to apply one of the greenhouse shading preparations available from garden centres to the outside of the windows.

Further reading

Temporary Use of Liquefied Petroleum Gas Heaters in Schools, HSE 1986
Guidelines for Environmental Design and Fuel Conservation in Educational Buildings, Design Note 17, DES 1981

The Education (School Premises) Regulations 1981

These regulations, made under the Education Act 1944, apply to schools maintained by a local education authority, including voluntary aided and voluntary controlled schools. They spell out the minimum standards for school premises in respect of accommodation, washrooms, provision of rooms for headteachers, heating, lighting, the thermal environment, water supplies, and playing fields.

Various improvements in provision introduced in this legislation were subject to a time delay until September 1991 to give LEAs an opportunity to implement them. However, the Education (School Premises) Amendment Regulations 1990 amended the deadline to September 1996.

Although some of the matters covered by these regulations are welfare provisions the Health and Safety Executive is not responsible for the enforcement of the Education Act or associated legislation.

Washrooms — pupils

The minimum provision of "washrooms" is specified in detail. Washrooms are defined as rooms having wash basins and sanitary fittings.

In primary/nursery schools there should be at least one sanitary fitting and wash basin for every 10 pupils under five years old, and one for every 20 pupils of five and older, numbers rounded up to the nearest whole even number. In no case should there be less than four fittings/basins provided. For pupils under five there must also be one deep sink for every 40 pupils, again rounded up to the nearest multiple of 40.

In secondary schools there should be at least one sanitary fitting for every 20 pupils, and there should be two wash basins for every three sanitary fittings.

In special schools the required provision is one sanitary fitting and wash basin for every 10 pupils, again with a minimum number of four and with pupil numbers rounded up.

In day schools not more than two-thirds of fittings in boys' washrooms will be urinals.

In boarding schools the minimum provision is one water closet for every five pupils. Wash basins must be provided on the following basis:

(a) one for every three pupils up to 60 pupils
(b) one for every four pupils for the next 40 pupils
(c) one for every additional five pupils.

Regulation 26 specifies that washbasins shall be provided with warm water at a temperature not exceeding 43.5°C. (In a tragic case in May 1991 an 11-year-old pupil with mental disabilities died at a school run by a charity. The boy ran himself a bath of scalding hot water and climbed in. The verdict of the Coroner's Court was death due to lack of care.)

Washrooms—staff

Regulation 11 requires that separate provision is made for male and female staff, and that staff provision must be separate from that made for pupils. Unfortunately there is no scale of provision laid down. In the absence of a precise standard the usual practice is to "borrow" and apply the levels specified in the Sanitary Accommodation Regulations 1964 which were made under the Offices, Shops and Railway Premises Act 1963. A scale of one water closet per 15 workers applies. The problem is that, whereas office workers can "spend a penny" whenever they want to, teachers cannot. Hence the undignified queues seen in many schools at breaktimes. (This problem will be largely solved by legislation to be implemented in existing schools by 1 January 1996 (see "Workplace Health, Safety and Welfare) Regulations 1992") (W(HSW)R).)

From 1 September 1991 (amended to 1 September 1996) changing accommodation and showers should be available for staff engaged in physical education in schools where there are pupils who have attained the age of eight years. However, the W(HSW)R, which take precedence over these regulations, require such provision no later than 1 September 1996 in existing schools and immediately in new premises.

Drinking water (R.26)

Schools shall have a "wholesome" supply of water for domestic purposes which, so far as is reasonably practicable, will be drawn from the mains.

Staffrooms

Regulation 13(3) says that every school must include accommodation for teachers for the "purposes of work (otherwise than in teaching accommodation) and for social purposes". Although the quality and size of such accommodation is not specified it is implied that it should be reasonable in both respects. DES Building Bulletin No. 25, 1965, while not prescribing fixed standards for staffrooms does attempt to "look critically at accommodation for teaching staff and ask what ought to be provided".

There has been some debate about the need for DES premises regulations given the introduction of the W(HSW)R. It is understood that the DES will be issuing new regulations towards the end of 1993. It is anticipated that they will concentrate on provisions for pupils, an area not covered by W(HSW)R.

Further reading

The Education (School Premises) Regulations 1981 (SI 909), HMSO
The Education (School Premises) Amendment Regulations 1990 (SI 2351)
Guidance for Environmental Design etc in Educational Buildings, Design Note 17, DES 1981

Chapter 15
School Kitchens

Catering staff are perhaps 20 times more likely to suffer injury at work than are teachers. Their working environment is hazardous. They are required to work to meet deadlines, kitchen equipment is often old and poorly maintained and staff training is not always as thorough as it should be.

Examination of the accident statistics for a large LEA shows that in a typical year 30 per cent of all staff accidents occurred in school kitchens despite catering staff being only a small proportion of total staff numbers. Over a third of these accidents were slips and falls, 17 per cent were burns and scalds, 16 per cent were cuts, 10 per cent were lifting injuries, the balance arising from the use of cleaning materials, collisions with furniture and doors, etc.

In 1985 this LEA's catering service estimated that slips and falls injuries in its 800 kitchens were costing at least £600,000 per year in lost staff time, quite apart from the pain and suffering to the people involved.

If pupils are allowed into school kitchens it must always be under the closest supervision.

It is important that kitchen staff are fully integrated into the health and safety arrangements of the school. In particular they should be represented on the school safety committee and should be involved in fire drills (see "Fire").

Slips and Falls

Many floors that have a reasonable slip resistance when dry become dangerous when wet or greasy. Kitchen flooring materials often seem to

179

have been specified with only "cleanability" in mind, without consideration of the safety of workers using the area. Quarry tiles are reasonably safe when dry and clean but that is not a condition that is easy to maintain in a busy kitchen. (Cleaning quarry tiles with alkali detergents has been found to have a glazing effect over a period of time, further reducing slip resistance.) Inadequate ventilation, especially during the winter months, causes condensation problems that no amount of wiping of floors will overcome.

Catering workers are normally expected to wear "sensible" shoes for work. Employers may find that to provide shoes with a high slip resistance in wet conditions will prove to be a cost effective investment, especially in those kitchens where the floors are less than ideal.

If it is not possible to replace unsatisfactory floors immediately considerable improvements can be made by heating the kitchen adequately in the winter months and by ensuring that there is sufficient ventilation. (A common situation is that the only available ventilation is excessive. The fans are unduly noisy and the kitchen becomes cold, so the system is not switched on.)

In areas where slips can have serious consequences (eg around sterilisers) the use of non-slip tape on the floor should be considered. The cook in charge must ensure that every effort is made to keep floors clean and dry. Any spillage of food or liquid must be cleaned up immediately, and the final floor washing at the end of the day must be organised so that no one needs to walk on wet areas.

In the event of ice and snow the need to keep access to the kitchen, and from the kitchen to dustbins, in a safe condition must not be forgotten. (For specific legal requirements, from 1 January 1996 in existing schools, see Regulation 12 Workplace (Health, Safety and Welfare) Regulations 1992.)

Gas Appliances

Gas appliances require regular servicing to ensure that they remain in a safe condition and that they are operating efficiently. There should be an annual check made by a competent engineer (eg from a company registered with CORGI, the Confederation for the Registration of Gas Installers).

Many ovens used in school kitchens are not equipped with a pilot/flame failure device. A number of accidents have occurred when the person lighting an oven has turned on the gas and waited too long before applying a lighted match. Loss of hair and burns to the face and arms usually result. The oven door should be opened and the match prepared for lighting before the gas is turned on.

Food Preparation Machines

S.19 of the Offices, Shops and Railway Premises Act 1963, which covers canteen kitchens, states that no one may be put to work on "specified dangerous machines" unless fully instructed in the dangers and precautions to be observed. Furthermore, every person must receive sufficient training in work at the machine, or at the very least, work under competent and experienced supervision. The dangerous machines referred to include the following:

(a) powered worm type mincing machines
(b) powered rotary knife bowl type chopping machines
(c) powered dough brakes and mixers
(d) powered mixing machines when used with attachments for mincing, slicing, chipping, or any other cutting operation, or for crumbling
(e) powered vegetable slicing machines
(f) potato chipping machines, whether or not powered
(g) circular blade slicing machines, whether or not powered.

The guarding on some types of commercially available catering machines is not foolproof, and the safety of users has to rely on their training and skill. Particular care is necessary when cleaning the blades of slicing machines (eg bacon slicers) and when feeding food into machine hoppers. (For details of legal requirements from 1 January 1997 see Provision and Use of Work Equipment Regulations 1992.)

Kitchens tend to be damp places and dampness can significantly increase the risk of death occurring as a result of an electrical shock. Much electrically powered catering equipment is metal cased and if an internal fault occurs the case may become live at a lethal voltage unless it is effectively earthed. Effective earthing relies on the cable being in good condition, the plug being properly made off and the building's wiring being in good order. Given the low cost involved, the increased risk because of damp conditions and the likely severe consequences, it would be difficult to argue that the provision of a residual current device in the mains supply circuit to the kitchens would not be reasonably practicable (see "Electrical Safety").

Skin Problems

Irritant contact dermatitis is a frequent but preventable problem among catering staff. Less common, but more serious, are cases of allergic contact dermatitis (see "Dermatitis").

While simple precautions at work can virtually eliminate the problem, it is also necessary to ensure that staff understand the need to take appropriate care of their hands at home. It is suspected that a proportion of cases of apparent occupational dermatitis that occur in kitchens are actually caused at home and that work just exacerbates the condition. Any activity that removes the natural oils from the skin and/or affects its pH balance is likely to cause problems. If, for example, hands are immersed in detergent laced water and removed and dried without first rinsing them the detergent remains in the pores and the condition known as "washday red hands" is a distinct possibility. (This is the first stage of irritant contact dermatitis.) Even regular exposure to plain hot water for an hour or so may cause skin damage.

To avoid these problems the following steps should be taken:

(a) when working with any liquid—
  (i) products should be diluted to the strength recommended by the manufacturer
  (ii) wear impervious gloves with sleeves long enough to prevent the liquid getting inside
  (iii) if it is not practical to wear gloves for a task a barrier cream specifically designed for wet work should be applied to the hands
  (iv) if detergent, etc gets onto the skin it should be rinsed off with clean water and carefully dried.
(b) at the end of each working day the hands should be washed thoroughly with mild soap and water and carefully rinsed and dried. A skin conditioning cream should be applied. It will be found that wearing impervious gloves will irritate some pre-existing skin conditions.

Alkali substances such as bleach and oven cleaners will adversely affect the pH of the skin, as well as causing surface damage, and particular care is needed when they are used. Some detergents, soaps and disinfectants can sensitise a genetically predisposed worker and allergic contact dermatitis results. In such cases the only solution is for the substance in question to be totally avoided and this usually means the sufferer has to find a different type of employment.

When recruiting kitchen staff it is sensible to avoid employing anyone who has a previous history of skin problems.

Lifting and Handling

Injuries to kitchen staff arising from lifting and handling activities are common. The requirements of the Manual Handling Operations Regulations 1992 will have particular relevance in kitchens, especially in respect of the use of sack barrows and trolleys, the size and packages and the organisation of store rooms. (See "Manual Handling".)

Dining Areas

Slips and falls are a frequent cause of injury in dining areas where food and liquids have been spilt on the floor. A system should be devised to ensure that such spills are cleaned up as soon as they occur.

Fire and First Aid

Every kitchen must be provided with a first aid box (see "First Aid") and with appropriate means of dealing with small fires. Typical provision of fire extinguishing equipment is:

(a) a fire blanket, and
(b) a 2.5 kg CO_2 extinguisher, or
(c) a 2 kg dry powder extinguisher.

The fire prevention officer from the fire brigade will usually make recommendations on the necessary level of provision and give instruction to staff on the use of hand fire appliances. Instruction for kitchen staff in the safe and effective use of fire blankets is especially important.

Food Safety Law

Food Safety Act 1990

This legislation was designed to strengthen consumer protection and to combat the incidence of food poisoning cases arising from the consumption of food prepared and sold on non-domestic premises. It covers all parts of the food chain from manufacturers to retailers. Enforcement is the responsibility of environmental health officers (EHOs) employed by local authorities.

It applies to school kitchens and canteens, whether or not they are operated for profit, to school tuck shops and to occasional events where, perhaps, food is prepared by pupils, parents and teachers for sale to the public. It also applies where schools purchase food ingredients for home economics work if pupils subsequently pay for them.

S.7 makes it an offence to render food injurious to health by adding or subtracting harmful ingredients, articles or substances, or by subjecting it to a process or treatment.

This covers cases where foreign bodies (such as parts of food preparation machines, cigarette ends and first aid dressings) get into food. It also covers treatments such as adding curry powder to unfit food to mask its flavour, and inadequate processes such as the undercooking of chicken, if they result in food injurious to health being sold. The person responsible being unaware of the consequences of their action is not a defence.

Under s.8 it is an offence to sell, advertise for sale, possess for the purpose of selling, or to prepare food not complying with food safety requirements. It is also illegal to pass such food to someone else to be sold. Food will not comply with safety requirements if it has been rendered injurious to health as described in s.7, if it is unfit for human consumption, or if it is so contaminated that it would be unreasonable for it to be used for human consumption.

Ss.14 and 15 require that food is of the nature, substance and quality demanded by the purchaser, and that labelling must accurately describe the nature and quantity of the food in question.

S.21 provides that in the event of a prosecution it will be a defence to be able to show that all reasonable precautions were taken and "due diligence" was exercised to avoid the commission of the offence.

In other words it is accepted that there can never be an absolute certainty that defective food will not be sold but the seller should always be able to demonstrate that "reasonable precautions" and "due diligence" were in place.

EHOs retain the powers of inspection and seizure of suspect food specified in previous legislation. In addition they can now serve improvement and prohibition notices. Penalties on conviction are similar to those applying under the Health and Safety at Work, etc Act 1974.

The Food Premises (Registration) Regulations 1991

These require that premises are registered with the local authority if food is sold there on any five days in any five consecutive weeks. (In county schools kitchens may have been registered *en bloc*. EHOs visiting such kitchens should be informed of any other food retailing activities carried on in the school.) Failure to register premises can result in a fine of up to £400. (Registration involves completion of a simple form. It is recommended that proof of posting the form (eg a certificate of posting) is retained, or acknowledgement of receipt is obtained from the local authority.)

Food Hygiene (General) Regulations 1970

These regulations, as amended by the Food Hygiene (Amendment) Regulations 1990 and 1991, spell out detailed requirements in respect of food premises, equipment, personal hygiene of staff, storage of food, washing facilities and sanitary conveniences.

The situation of and condition of food premises must not be such as to create a risk of contamination of food. Walls, ceilings, doors, floors and all other parts, must be kept clean and maintained in good order. Construction should be such as to avoid, as far as is possible, infestations by birds, rodents and insects. Lighting and ventilation must be adequate and the water supply clean and wholesome. Food rooms must not be used for sleeping and, usually, no room which communicates directly with a sleeping place may be used for handling open food.

Equipment with which food comes into contact must be kept clean and in good condition. It must be possible to clean it thoroughly. Equipment should be such as to prevent, so far as is reasonably practicable, the absorption of matter and any risk of contamination of food.

Food handlers in kitchens must wear clean, washable overalls. Other clothing and footwear may only be kept in a room where food is handled if it is in closed lockers or cupboards. Food handlers must keep themselves and their overalls clean. They must refrain from using tobacco in rooms where there is open food and from spitting. They must cover with a suitable waterproof dressing any cut or abrasion to exposed skin.

If persons employed to handle food become aware that they are either suffering from, or are carriers of, paratyphoid or any other salmonella infection, typhoid, dysentery or a staphylococcal infection they must immediately inform the headteacher, who will advise the school doctor. (see "Infectious Diseases" and "Food Poisoning").

A first aid box must be provided in a readily accessible position and contain individually wrapped waterproof sterile adhesive dressings (see "First Aid").

Food must not be allowed to come into contact with any article, container or wrapping material that might cause contamination. Live animals or poultry must not be allowed in food preparation areas.

Kitchen areas must be provided with conveniently positioned wash-hand basins. Each basin must be supplied with hot and cold water, soap (or a suitable substitute), a nail brush and means of hand drying. Basins provided for hand washing must not be used for any other purpose.

Sanitary conveniences provided for kitchen staff must not be in areas directly communicating with food handling areas. They must be kept clean and in good order, and "Wash your hands" notices must be displayed in prominent positions.

The Food Hygiene (Amendment) Regulations 1990

These regulations specify requirements for the storage of cooked food. Hot food must be maintained at a temperature above 63°C and cold food below 8°C. The foods concerned are:

(a) smoked or cured fish★
(b) cut or sliced, smoked or cured meat★
(c) pâtés and soft cheeses★
(d) cooked products containing meat, fish, eggs, cheese, cereals, pulses or vegetables★
(e) cooked pies, pasties and sausage rolls (unless intended to be consumed no later than the day after preparation)
(f) salads, cream cakes and some dairy deserts
(g) certain meat and fish pastries
(h) sandwiches and rolls containing fish, eggs, cheese, etc (where not to be consumed within 24 hours★).

(From 1 April 1993 those foods marked * must be stored below 5°C.)

Hot food to be eaten within two hours of preparation or cold food to be eaten within four hours of preparation are exempted from these requirements. Food may not be displayed on self-service counters for longer than four hours. Certain exemptions also apply where food is being defrosted. For detailed information consult the local authority EHO.

Written arrangements

While the food hygiene standards in most school kitchens are superior to those found in local commercial undertakings even the best run establishment can experience an outbreak of food poisoning due to a momentary lapse on someone's part. It is recommended that a short document spelling out the school's arrangements for food safety be prepared and appended to the school health and safety statement, and be displayed in the kitchen.

It should spell out the following:

(a) who has overall and local responsibility for catering areas
(b) the frequency of hygiene inspections
(c) cleaning schedules
(d) arrangements for equipment maintenance
(e) dealing with infestations of insects, rodents and birds (a common cause of prosecutions under food safety law)
(f) the ill-health of food handlers reporting system
(g) arrangements for induction and periodic staff training
(h) arrangements for monitoring food temperatures (if applicable)
(i) the responsibilities of food handlers in respect of their personal hygiene.

The local authority EHOs are usually willing to give specific advice on any matters relating to food hygiene.

Courses in basic food hygiene for food handlers, and more advanced courses for supervisors and managers, are run in many parts of the country. The EHOs should be able to give advice about the availability of such courses locally.

Further reading

Catering Safety: Food Preparation Machinery, HSG 35 HSE, HMSO
Health Service Catering: Safety at Work, DHSS Leaflets Unit, PO Box 21,
Stanmore, Middlesex HA7 1AY

Risks à la Carte: Safety Representatives' Guides to Catering Hazards, GMBATU, Thorne House, Ruxley Ridge, Claygate, Esher, Surrey
Catering, Croner (a loose-leaf book with bi-monthly updates covering all aspects of catering)
Health and Safety in Kitchens and Food Preparation Areas, HSG55, HSE, HMSO
Health Surveillance of Occupational Skin Disease, HMSO
Clean Food: A Food Handler's Guide, HMSO
The Food Safety Act 1990 and You, HM Government, 1992 (Available from Foodsense, London SE99 7TT)

Chapter 16

The Control of Substances Hazardous to Health (COSHH) Regulations 1988

These regulations, made under the Health and Safety at Work, etc Act 1974, came into effect on 1.10.89. They represent the most important steps towards protecting the health of people at work since the original Act.

Employers are now required to have a formal assessment made of the risks that might arise from the use at work of substances defined as hazardous to health. Precautions commensurate to the risk must be specified and implemented. Any mechanical measures (such as extraction systems, fume cupboards) used to control risks must be subject to periodic formal inspection, and records kept to prove that this requirement has been complied with. The regulations require that employees are fully briefed about any risks involved in the use of a substance and the measures necessary to counter them. Employees are required to make full and proper use of any protective equipment provided to protect their health, and to report immediately any defects in it to their employer. From 1.1.90 it is an offence for any substance defined as "hazardous to health" to be used at a place of work without a formal assessment having been made.

Substances "Hazardous to Health"

The regulations cover substances in the following categories:

(a) substances labelled by suppliers "very toxic", "toxic", "harmful", "corrosive" or "irritant"
(b) substances for which a maximum exposure is specified
(c) a micro-organism used at work that constitutes a hazard to health
(d) dust of any kind if it is present in substantial concentration in air
(e) any substance not included above which creates a comparable hazard to health.

Substances assigned a maximum exposure limit ((b) above) include hard wood dust, vinyl chloride, trichloroethylene 1,1,1 — Trichloroethane, man made mineral fibre, and formaldehyde.

Radioactive materials, lead and asbestos are covered by other specific legislation and are excluded from the COSHH Regulations, as are materials hazardous to health because of their flammable or explosive properties.

COSHH Regulations and Schools

At first glance the implications of these regulations for secondary schools are daunting. Hundreds of substances falling within the above definition are used in areas such as science, art and CDT, and require assessment. Strictly, the requirement is for an assessment to be made for a substance used in particular ways and in particular circumstances. If that substance is then to be used in a different way another assessment must be made. The vast majority of these substances, however, are used in small quantities, in a carefully prescribed way, and infrequently.

Secondary schools that are subscribers, either individually or through their LEA, to the Consortium of Local Education Authorities for the Provision of Science Services (CLEAPSS) will have been issued with sets of "Hazcards" covering all hazardous substances used in normal school science. The information given on these cards, when used in conjunction with recommended standard texts, constitute, in the view of the Education Safety Advisory Committee (ESAC) "suitable and sufficient assessments". CLEAPSS also provides a very efficient advice service to cover circumstances when it is proposed to use a substance or carry out an operation that is not covered in the recommended texts. For primary school science the CLEAPSS booklet LP5 *Safe Use of Household and Other Chemicals* is considered to constitute an adequate general assessment.

Unfortunately, such general assessments are not available for substances used in all other subjects, but CLEAPSS recently produced assessments for substances used in the CDT area, and these are available to their subscribers. Substances used in cleaning and maintenance of the premises must not be forgotten. In practice it is in these areas, where the exposure of staff to substances may be regular and significant, that the application of these regulations in schools is most relevant.

The Education Service Advisory Committee (ESAC) has published a booklet *COSHH Guidance for Schools*. It points out that when delegating the task of making assessments the employer must ensure that it is carried out by someone who is fully aware of the legal requirements, the approved code of practice, etc, and of how and where the product is used. That person will also need some knowledge of occupational health, or have access to informed advice so that suitable and sufficient assessments are made. Most LEAs employ people trained in occupational health and safety who can provide such advice, but independent schools may need either to buy in expert assistance or arrange for members of staff to receive appropriate training. Apart from any problems likely to be encountered during normal usage, consideration must be given to risks arising during storage and if spillages occur.

Manufacturers and suppliers of products used at a place of work are legally required (s.6(4) Health and Safety at Work, etc Act 1974, amended by the Consumer Protection Act 1987) to provide customers with a product data sheet. (The Health and Safety Executive booklet *Substances for Use at Work: The Provision of Information* HS(G)27 gives advice on how to interpret such information.) These provide information and advice on which an assessment can be based. If the information supplied is unclear, or if it does not appear to cover the usage envisaged, the supplier/manufacturer should be asked for clarification. Enquiries should be made to establish whether there is a less dangerous substitute that could be used instead of the product in question, or if it could be purchased in a less dangerous form (eg acid may be being purchased in a concentrated form and diluted for use, when purchase in a diluted form eliminates much of the danger in storage and use).

While most assessments will be written out in some detail, occasionally this will not be necessary. For example, bottles of Tipp-Ex solvent are labelled "harmful" and as such require that an assessment is made. The assessment may well be that the risk from its use does not warrant further action. A note should, however, be made to that effect.

Safety representatives must be consulted about the way that these regulations are to be implemented, and they should be provided with copies of all written assessments relating to substances used by the staff that they represent. They are expected to encourage cooperation between the employer and employees in the promotion and development of measures to ensure the health of employees, and to check on the effectiveness of such measures.

Arrangements must be made to ensure that any future introduction of a new substance or a change in the use of an existing substance is not permitted until any necessary assessments have been made. This might be achieved by requiring staff to seek authorisation from the head of department in a secondary school or the headteacher in primary schools. Details of the system adopted should be spelled out in the school's written health and safety arrangements.

The approach adopted by one LEA has been to identify all hazardous substances used on its premises and to have assessments made centrally. Officers qualified in occupational health and safety produced some 50 assessments which were then forwarded to the establishments where they were applicable, with detailed instructions for implementation. Many were general assessments, covering a number of substances, while others were specific. Those assessments issued to schools were:

(a) cleaning materials
(b) soft soldering
(c) small scale use of white spirit
(d) photographic chemicals
(e) wood dust
(f) teaching of science in secondary schools
(g) teaching of science in primary schools
(h) aerosol fixative
(i) washing up liquids and cleaning materials used in kitchens
(j) dilute hydrochloric and sulphuric acid used in non-science areas
(k) small scale work with epoxy metal paste
(l) small scale work with glass reinforced plastic
(m) aerosol foam cleaner
(n) aerosol adhesives—spray mount and photo mount
(o) substances used in pottery
(p) small scale use of adhesives
(q) trichloroisocyanuric acid (swimming pools)
(r) sodium hypochlorite (swimming pools)
(s) hydrochloric acid (swimming pools)
(t) substances used in screen printing

(u) substances used in small scale offset litho printing
(v) eight individual assessments covering pesticides and herbicides used by school gardeners and a few schools (Gramoxone, Turbair Permethrin, Turbair Resmethrin Extra, Malathion, Reglone, Turbair Systemic Insecticide, Grazone 90 and Roundup).

Two examples of hazard assessments follow. The first is in respect of wood dust and is general in that it does not differentiate between different types of wood. All wood dust is assumed to have "worst case" potential. The second example is in respect of cleaning materials. A general assessment was made because the risks involved are not sufficient to warrant individual assessments, and adopting a "worst case" approach for all products provided best protection for staff without creating unnecessary confusion.

Example 1—Wood Dust

Exbridge School for Boys
Control of Substances Hazardous to Health Regulations 1988

Head of CDT
You are required to ensure so far as is reasonably practicable:
(a) that any employee exposed to wood dust is informed of the hazards and the precautions specified in this document
(b) that the precautions are taken and that the control measures are used and maintained
(c) that the specified personal protective equipment is used and maintained. (It will be visually checked for condition each term and a formal record kept to prove that this has been done.)

Members of staff exposed to wood dust
Regulation 8 requires you to use any personal protective equipment, extraction ventilation and dust collection systems provided to protect your health when machining wood. You are required by law to report immediately to the HOD any defect in that equipment or those systems.

Assessment of health risk (Regulation 6) wood dust, and dusts from chipboard and MDF boards
Regulation 2 defines "dust of any kind, when present in substantial concentration in air" as a substance hazardous to health. Hard wood dust is listed in schedule 1 to the regulations and has a long term exposure limit of 5 mg m^3.
Wood dust gives rise to various harmful effects, the nature of which depend

193

on the constituents of the wood in question. Most commercially available woods produce dust that is harmful in some respect. Pine, afromosia, mahogany, boxwood, chestnut, cedar, iroko, beech, ramin, spruce, teak, yew, cherry and oak are among those woods known to cause dermatitis, conjunctivitis, rhinitis and asthma, while elm, plane, ash and maple are known to cause dermatitis. Given the difficulty of identifying many woods, especially when used in plywood, and the fact that the effects of some exotic woods are not known, all wood dust will be treated as equally harmful. Wood dust produces several direct effects including eye irritation and irritation of the upper respiratory tract and lungs, with initial symptoms such as sweating, coughing and hoarseness. Chronic irritation may produce permanent changes in these tissues. It also produces allergic reactions in susceptible individuals (asthma, rhinitis) and skin disorders characterised by itching, dermatitis or eczma and nettle rash.

In industrial conditions some wood dust has proved to be carcinogenic.

It is most unlikely that the concentration of wood dust in air in the school workshop would, when averaged over an eight hour period, reach the long term exposure limit. Nevertheless, high levels of exposure can arise for short periods, particularly when powered sanding of wood takes place. Such exposure is undesirable and, in the case of persons genetically predisposed to allergies, may be sufficient to trigger asthmatic and dermatitic conditions.

Control of exposure to wood dust (Regulation 7)

No powered sanding will be carried out indoors unless the machine is fitted with dust collection or extraction facilities.

The circular saw and planer/thicknesser must be fitted with extraction facilities unless use is intermittent.

Where the dust collection or extraction facilities are not effective in controlling dust, respiratory and eye protection will be worn by everyone in the area.

For persons regularly employed in such circumstances the recommended respirator is: PNUE-SEAL DUST RESPIRATOR.

For pupils and other persons occasionally so exposed satisfactory protection will be given by: 3M's DUST MASKS.

Eye protection will be goggles, grade 1 Impact and Dust.

Dust collection or extraction is not a practicable proposition where the wood lathes are concerned. Dust production must therefore be minimised by using, so far as possible, chisels and gouges rather than scrapers. Scrapers will be kept sharp so that they pare rather than abrade the surface. Abrasives will not be used to shape a workpiece. Their use will be restricted to further refining a good finish produced with the tools. Eye and respiratory protection, as specified above, will be worn when using the lathes.

To reduce the possibility of dermatitis, wood dust must be kept, so far as is possible, off the skin. Clothing should be selected with this in mind (eg long sleeved with tight cuffs and buttoned to the neck). All exposed skin must be washed with soap and water as soon as possible after work is finished.

Maintenance and testing of control measures (Regulation 9)
The extraction, ventilation and dust collection facilities will be formally inspected for efficient operation every 14 months. Records will be kept by the HOD of these inspections.

Health problems
Any employees exposed to wood dusts who suspect that they may be experiencing any of the health problems described in this assessment should:

(a) see their general practitioner, explaining the nature of the work that they do
(b) advise the HOD.

Information, instructions and training (Regulation 12)
All employees who might be exposed to wood dusts must be given sufficient information, instruction and/or training in the hazards arising so that they know:

(a) the risks to health created
(b) the precautions that must be taken.

Example 2—Cleaning Materials

St Mary's Primary School
Control of Substances Hazardous to Health Regulations 1988

The Caretaker
You are required to ensure so far as is reasonably practicable:

(a) that cleaning staff are informed of the hazards and the necessary precautions described in this assessment
(b) that the precautions are taken
(c) that the specified personal protective equipment is kept available, is maintained in good condition and is used. (You will carry out a formal check of its condition twice per term and you will keep a record to show that this has been done.)

Cleaners
You are legally required to make full and proper use of the personal protective

equipment provided to protect your health. You are also required to report immediately any defect in that equipment to the caretaker.

Assessment of health risks (Regulation 6)
The products used in school for routine cleaning do present a few health hazards but these are readily countered by adopting simple precautions and strictly complying with the manufacturer's instructions. Those products designed to dissolve grease will also readily remove natural oils from skin. Bleach is an alkali solution that will affect the pH balance of the skin, while acidic descalers may cause superficial surface damage.

Such damage may cause irritant contact dermatitis and inflammation, with possible blistering, affecting the areas where the substance has been in contact with the skin.

People who suffer with hay fever, asthma and other allergies are liable to become sensitised to substances such as detergents, soaps and disinfectants. If this happens subsequent contact with the substance will result in a skin reaction, perhaps affecting the whole body. This condition is called allergic contact dermatitis.

Lavatory cleaners, oven cleaners and descaling liquids may cause permanent damage to the surface of the eye if prolonged contact occurs.

Control of exposure (Regulation 7)
To avoid such problems the following precautions will be taken by cleaning staff:

(a) ensure that products are diluted to the strength recommended by the manufacturer

(b) for all wet work you will wear impervious gloves with long sleeves (Gloves must be regularly inspected for damage and discarded as soon as they become unserviceable.)

(c) if it is not practical to wear gloves for any wet work a barrier cream, designed for wet work, will be supplied by the caretaker and must be used

(d) if substances inadvertently come into contact with the skin, wash the area in clean water and dry thoroughly

(e) never mix products (If bleach comes into contact with an acid such as descalers or lavatory cleaners, significant quantities of chlorine, a gas that irritates the lungs will be released. Acid descalers must never be used on the swimming pool surrounds while the pool is in use because chlorine will be released from the water and may affect persons swimming.)

(f) when using oven cleaners, and any other product where the manufacturer so specifies, eye protection will be worn

(g) if any cleaning products get into the eyes they must be thoroughly flushed with water for at least 10 minutes and medical assistance sought

(h) at the end of each work session hands must be thoroughly washed, rinsed

196

and dried (Skin conditioning cream, supplied by the caretaker, will be applied to hands and forearms.)

Health problems
If members of the cleaning staff experience any of the health problems described in this assessment they should:

(a) see their doctor and explain the nature of their work
(b) tell the caretaker, who will then advise the headteacher.

Consortium of Local Education Authorities for the Provision of Science Services

LEAs or individual schools wishing to use the consortium's services should write to: The Director, School Science Service, Brunel University, Uxbridge UB8 3PH.

Further reading

Control of Substances Hazardous to Health: Approved Code of Practice and Regulations, HMSO
COSHH Assessments. A Step by Step Guide to Assessments and the Skills Needed For It, HSE
COSHH: Guidance for Schools, ESAC, HMSO
EH 40/92 (revised annually) Occupational Exposure Limits, HSE, HMSO
Substances for Use at Work: The Provision of Information, HS(G)27, HSE
Houston, Dr. A *Dangerous Chemicals: Emergency First Aid Guide*, Croner 1990
Warren, P J and Potts, J M *Dangerous Chemicals: Emergency Spillage Guide*, Croner 1990
COSHH in the Production of Pottery, ACOP, HMSO 1990
Hardwood Dust, IND(S) 21(L) REV, HSE
COSHH and s.6 of Health and Safety at Work Act, IND(G) 97(L), HSE
COSHH: Its Application in the Foundry, HMSO
COSHH: Subject Catalogue, HSE 1990

Chapter 17
Violence and Security

Staff working in schools are required to control large numbers of people, a tiny minority of whom may react to authority in a violent way. Serious physical injury resulting from such incidents is extremely rare but too many teachers suffer lesser injury, threats and abuse, and criminal damage to their property when carrying out their duties. Such problems do not only involve pupils. Occasionally parents threaten or assault staff, and trying to deal with intruders on school premises can involve some risk. Violence may also be suffered by staff attempting to prevent theft, particularly when taking or collecting cash from the bank.

In some schools such occurrences are unknown and most teachers will enjoy a trouble free career in this respect. The effects on those colleagues who are not so fortunate, however, can be extremely traumatic and can even result in their leaving the profession.

Employers have a duty of care towards their employees and are required to take all reasonable steps to protect them from danger. Discharge of this responsibility requires employers to analyse all likely sources of violence, to determine what reasonable measures can be taken to minimise risks, to put those measures into effect, to examine any subsequent cases to see whether any refinement of the arrangements are warranted, and to provide members of staff who have been subjected to violent behaviour with support and assistance.

Pupils

Where the large majority of normally well behaved pupils are concerned the only precautionary measure that can reasonably be taken against violent conduct is to ensure that they know that the consequences of such conduct would be severe. Ultimately the best defence is for the idea of violence towards staff to be unthinkable.

Where a pupil of known violent propensities is concerned the situation is different. If, for example, a pupil has been expelled from a school for violence towards staff and is then sent to another school it is necessary for all staff there who may come into contact with the pupil to be fully briefed. Depending on the circumstances of the case, special arrangements may be necessary for additional supervision. While the best interests of such a pupil must be protected this should not be done at the expense of the safety of staff.

Intruders

When strangers are found in the school or its grounds and cannot provide a valid reason for being there they should be politely asked to leave and be seen off the premises. Staff should not attempt to evict intruders by force. If intruders refuse to leave and/or if it is suspected that they have committed or were intending to commit a criminal offence the police should be summoned. Headteachers should lay down clear guidelines for staff about the circumstances which will require that the police be called.

Where intruders are a recurring problem, consideration should be given to the possibility of improving physical arrangements on the premises. This may include:

(a) limiting access to the site and to each building to one entry (but, of course, maintaining means of escape exits)
(b) use of low fencing to encourage visitors towards a reception point, perhaps near the school office (Clear signposting is also important.)
(c) providing a satisfactory means of communication between buildings and within buildings.

If vandalism by intruders out of school hours is a problem, and if the premises are overlooked by houses it may prove worthwhile to write to local residents asking for any suspicious activity to be reported to the police.

The local police will usually be willing to provide help and advice on any matters relating to the prevention of crime. They may also be prepared to give guidance to staff on the line of approach that is least likely to result in violence in confrontational situations.

Legal Action

Prior to 1982 trespass on local authority school premises was a civil law matter. S.40 of the Local Government (Miscellaneous Provisions) Act 1982 now enables the police to remove from local authority premises anyone who is not authorised to be there and who causes a nuisance or a disturbance. Under ss.4 and 5 of the Public Order Act 1986 the police have the powers to arrest anyone whose threatening, insulting or abusive words or behaviour give rise to fears of violence against a person or property. They can also arrest anyone whose disorderly conduct is likely to cause harassment, alarm or distress and who does not respond to their warning to stop.

S.40 provides for a fine on conviction of up to £100. Prosecutions may be brought by the local authority or by the police. The decision to prosecute under s.4 and s.5 of the Public Order Act 1986 is normally made by the Crown Prosecution Service on a police recommendation.

If the police are called to a school as a result of a serious physical assault they can arrest the perpetrator and take direct legal proceedings, provided the victim is prepared to sign the charge sheet and give evidence in court.

Individuals who have been assaulted may be able to bring a prosecution against their assailant. Some employers will provide legal advice in such circumstances, or advice can be obtained from a trade union or a private solicitor. Obtaining such advice before proceeding further is to be recommended. A person bringing a prosecution must be prepared to attend a magistrates' or juvenile court for the taking out of a summons, to have their name on the summons and subsequently to give evidence in court.

Handling Cash Safely

Thieves are often prepared to use violence towards staff when stealing money. This is a risk particularly when depositing or drawing cash from the bank, but care must also be taken when making up wage packets in offices and when counting cash raised at school functions.

When staff carry large amounts to or from the bank common sense precautions should be applied:

(a) if regular trips are made, vary the route used and the time of day
(b) exercise extra vigilance in the first and last 100 metres of the journey, when most robberies take place
(c) if possible the cash should be secreted about the person and an empty "sacrificial" bag or case carried
(d) if an attack takes place resistance should not be offered if there is any risk of injury.

At school functions several members of staff should accompany the cash to the room where it is to be counted. At least two people should lock themselves in the room while counting is carried out and together they should take the money to the school safe or the night facility at the bank.

When making up wage packets in offices the door should be kept locked. While this work is going on, care should be taken to avoid the cash being seen from corridor windows, etc.

Further reading

Crime Prevention in Schools, Building Bulletin No. 69, DES
Violence to Staff in the Education Sector, HMSO 1990

Chapter 18
Asbestos

In the early 1980s there was great public concern about the possible health effects of exposure to asbestos fibres in the environment. The effects of high exposures in mines and factories were well documented and, in the absence of any significant evidence either way, campaigners pressed the approach that if a large exposure created a large risk a small exposure meant a small risk. They considered that even a small risk was unacceptable and some schools suffered serious disruptions, with staff walkouts and parents not sending their children to school. A number of LEAs responded by allocating very large sums of money to programmes to remove all the material from school premises.

Asbestos is a term used to describe a number of different silicate minerals. The most important commercially used types are chrysotile ("white"), amosite ("brown") and crocidolite ("blue"), with white being by far the most common.

The Health Risk

Over a lifetime everyone breathes in quantities of various types of insoluble mineral dusts. Particles greater than 5 microns in size are effectively dealt with by the body's defence mechanisms but smaller particles lodge in the lung and cause fibrosis. This may be thought of as scarring and its effect is to interfere with the oxygen/blood interface and thereby reduce lung efficiency. Typically, we may experience a reduction of, say, 20 per cent in lung efficiency over a 70 year period, but as we can live comfortably with a 50 per cent reduction this effect is not significant. If, however, a person is occupationally exposed to high levels of respirable sized mineral dusts over a working life not only does the fibrosis become significant but because the defence mechanisms are continually overloaded the damage effect is disproportionally greater than that from a small exposure.

In the past coal miners have suffered silicosis, asbestos miners and people working with asbestos in factories have developed asbestosis, and masons have experienced "stone cutter's lung". These are among the various forms of pneumoconiosis and are crippling in that physical activity is restricted by the inability of the lungs to oxygenate sufficient blood to allow sustained energetic movement. Asbestosis is strictly an occupational rather than an environmental health problem. What has concerned campaigners, however, is that a high proportion of workers suffering with asbestosis develop lung cancer. Using a straight line extrapolation from high exposure/high risk to zero exposure/no risk they have suggested that low (environmental) exposures constitute a low risk of lung cancer. There is also a rare type of cancer, mesothelioma, associated with exposure to blue asbestos at environmental levels.

There has been a long debate about the validity of the straight line extrapolation approach. Recent research has tended to indicate that there may be a threshold of exposure below which no excess cases of lung cancer occur. For example, a report by the Ontario Royal Commission describes a five year study of a chrysotile mining town in Canada where environmental asbestos levels are between 250 and 500 times higher than other similar towns but even so no excess cases of lung cancer were found in people living there but not working in the mines. Research into the way that cells respond to asbestos fibres has greatly increased understanding of how cancer occurs in practice and has provided a possible explanation for the findings in other research of a threshold. There is also increasing evidence that suggests that asbestos will only cause lung cancer where asbestosis already exists. Nonetheless, there remain experts who argue that excess cases of lung cancer from low exposures do occur but that they are so small in number that they cannot be measured.

Asbestos in School Buildings

The import of crocidolite to the United Kingdom ceased in 1970 and since the mid-70s the importing of amosite and chrysotile has declined rapidly and significantly. Vigorous efforts have been made by manufacturers to find satisfactory substitutes and there is now no reason why new buildings should contain asbestos. In most existing schools, however, it is found in various forms:

(a) *Sprayed asbestos*

This is a mixture of about 85 per cent asbestos (usually crocidolite) and cement that was sprayed onto structural steelwork, ceilings, etc to give fire protection, thermal insulation and acoustic dampening. Its use ceased in 1974. It is a friable, easily damaged material which readily releases fibres if disturbed. It tends to deteriorate with age.

(b) *Insulating boards*

This is low to medium density sheet material containing between 20 per cent and 40 per cent asbestos (usually amosite). It was widely used as ceiling tiles, in partitions, door facings, porch linings and as a general building board. If painted and in good condition there is no fibre release. If the surface is abraded or the sheet is broken fibre release will occur. (NB: There are sheet materials that are very similar in appearance but which contain no asbestos. Expert examination of samples is necessary to determine the content.)

(c) *Lagging*

Asbestos has been extensively used in the past as an insulation material for pipes, boilers etc. For such purposes it was used in various forms. It was mixed with a plaster like material and directly applied, it was precast into half round pipe sections, and made into felt strips, tape, string, etc. Any type of asbestos, or mixtures of types, may have been employed. The likelihood of fibre release depends on the condition of the material. It represents a special problem in that it will be damaged and disturbed when maintenance work is carried out.

(d) *Asbestos cement sheet*

This is a compressed material made of cement and about 15 per cent chrysotile. It may be in a flat or corrugated sheet, or moulded into shapes to form guttering, flue pipes, etc. It is a high density material. Experiments carried out for the ILEA indicated that breaking sheets with a hammer did not release fibres but weathering and acidic rain will, over a period of years, cause the surface of roofs to deteriorate such that some release may occur.

It is difficult to believe in the light of current knowledge that the blanket decisions made by some LEAs 10 years ago to remove all asbestos from their buildings would be repeated today. The cost was extremely high (eg £750,000 in one school) and perhaps 85 per cent of the material removed constituted not the slightest hazard to anyone. The removal process unavoidably put the health of the contractors at some risk, no matter how much care was taken to minimise this.

A sensible approach is to identify those materials which might constitute a risk and to deal with them. All other asbestos-bearing materials should be regularly monitored to ensure that damage or deterioration does not occur and that any sealing remains effective.

Sprayed asbestos that shows any sign of damage or deterioration should be effectively sealed, enclosed or removed. If it is in a position subject to mechanical damage it should be removed as a matter of priority.

Insulating boards should be sealed with a suitable paint. If they are in locations where they may be abraded or damaged they should either be protected by panelling or removed.

Asbestos cement materials within buildings should be kept painted. A careful watch should be kept where it is used externally and surface sealants applied if any deterioration becomes apparent.

The safe removal of asbestos is a highly specialised operation. Work should so far as is possible only be carried out during holiday periods, with air tests being made to ensure that no contamination remains before the area is reoccupied. The results of these tests must be given to safety representatives. It is important that such works are only entrusted to competent, experienced licensed contractors.

The need periodically to carry out maintenance work on pipes and boilers means that asbestos-bearing lagging will be subject to damage and disturbance. This may put the health of maintenance contractors at risk and licensing requirements may cause delays to the work. The Asbestos (Licensing) Regulations 1983 prohibit work with asbestos insulation and coatings by anyone not holding a licence granted by the Health and Safety Executive (HSE) unless the work takes less than two hours in any week and 28 days' notice has been given in writing prior to commencement of work. Work is defined as the repairing, removal or disturbance of asbestos insulation or coatings. Any unexpected and urgent repairs to, say, asbestos lagged pipes can present problems. (The HSE may be prepared to waive the 28 day notice period in special cases.) The early planned replacement of asbestos lagging with alternative materials is indicated.

When any immediate hazards have been eliminated school management and safety representatives should agree arrangements to ensure the continuing avoidance of any possible risk to health from those asbestos-bearing materials remaining on the premises. These arrangements should cover:

(a) the identification of all remaining asbestos-bearing materials, the making of a formal record and the caretaker and safety representative being provided with copies of the records

(b) regular inspections being made to ensure that encapsulating materials remain in good condition

(c) the caretaker ensuring that any contractors intending to carry out work in areas where there are asbestos-bearing materials are warned and, if the work is more than minor and may result in fibre release, that it is carried out while the premises are unoccupied

(d) contractors thoroughly cleaning up and removing any debris, etc that might contain asbestos fibres and, if there is any possibility of significant contamination, testing for fibres in air before reoccupation of the area by staff and pupils is permitted.

A standard was devised by the ILEA to be used when determining whether areas were safe for reoccupation in such cases. For an area to be considered clear the average of the air test readings taken could not exceed 0.01 fibres per millilitre of air.

Further reading

Report of the Royal Commission on matters of Health and Safety Arising From the Use of Asbestos in Ontario, Toronto 1984, Ontario Ministry of the Attorney General

Encyclopaedia of Occupational Health and Safety, 3rd edition, International Labour Office, Geneva 1983. (Volume 1 pages 195–197.)

Asbestos and You, IND(G) 17(L) HSE

The Control of Asbestos at Work Regulations 1987 (SI 2115), HMSO

The Asbestos (Licensing) Regulations 1983 (SI 1649), HMSO

Asbestos Materials in Buildings, Department of the Environment 1983

Vacuum Cleaners for Use with Asbestos, HSE 1984

A Guide to the Asbestos (Licensing) Regulations 1983, HS(R) 19, HMSO

Chapter 19
Work Experience

Encouraged by educational developments such as the Technical and Vocational Education Initiative (TVEI), schools are increasingly arranging work experience placements for their pupils. While pupils are engaged on such activities the school remains *in loco parentis*. The teachers responsible for such placements also have a duty under s.7 Health and Safety at Work, etc Act to ensure, so far as is reasonable, that their "acts or omissions" do not affect the health and safety of these pupils.

Various stories, apocryphal it is to be hoped, are heard of pupils being sent out to find their own placements without any check being made on the suitability of the workplace.

The Health and Safety (Training for Employment) Regulations 1990 have been made to extend to school-age pupils on work experience placements the same protection as is enjoyed by employees under health and safety legislation.

Teachers responsible for arranging work placements are not likely to be experts in industrial health and safety but they are expected to take reasonable measures to protect the health and safety of pupils. These will include visiting the workplace in question, assessing its suitability and being aware of the considerable legislation which prohibits persons under 18 years of age from carrying out various activities.

Employers should provide appropriate training for teachers expected to carry out these tasks.

Assessing the Suitability of a Workplace

Responsible employers will respect a thorough, professional approach on the part of the teacher.

It is essential that potential workplaces are visited. Visits provide an opportunity to explore all aspects of work experience with the employer, including health and safety. Through discussion it will be possible to form a clear picture of the requirements and expectations of both parties and to decide whether they can be met. The teacher should ask to see the area of work where the pupil would be based and to be allowed to talk to the supervisor and other employees working there. Their attitude towards health and safety is perhaps the most important factor in determining suitability or otherwise.

When looking at the workplace the teacher should consider the physical environment, evidence of safety awareness and attitudes to health and safety. Most potential placements will be neither very bad nor very good but ultimately it is necessary to be satisfied that the pupil will be reasonably safe there. If there should be any doubt it is wise not to proceed further.

Schools also have a responsibility to brief employers about the pupil. They need to know about any disability such as epilepsy, asthma and skin allergies, as well as any foreseeable difficulties in understanding instructions, whether through language difficulties or poor comprehension of written or oral instructions. Teachers need to consider whether a pupil has sufficient maturity and common sense, and is physically capable, of working safely in the environment in question.

Preparing for Work Experience

Pupils need to be fully briefed about the general rules governing health and safety at work. Their responsibility to themselves and others should be strongly emphasised. A number of publications, listed below, are available and should be used to reinforce the briefing. Pupils should be provided with the school telephone number and be instructed to use it if they are asked to do anything that they feel might be dangerous.

Monitoring Placements

Teachers should monitor the safety of pupils on placement, if possible by visiting to see them at work. Feedback from pupils after the placement should also be used to build up a list of suitable workplaces for future use.

Insurance

If pupils are placed at workplaces where the employer's liability insurance cover does not extend to them and they suffer a serious injury they would have to seek compensation from the employer. In the case of a small company this may mean bankruptcy and little or no compensation. It may be possible for the employer's liability cover to be extended to the pupils. Some companies will have public liability insurance which may cover pupils on placements but voluntary organisations and small family businesses may have neither employer's nor public liability insurance.

Where an employer or organisation does not hold and is unwilling to obtain appropriate insurance cover it is recommended that pupils are not sent there.

Some LEAs and schools take out a personal accident insurance policy covering pupils on work experience placements. If, say, a pupil is totally disabled in an accident whilst on work experience, compensation can normally only be obtained if either the school or the employer has been negligent or there was a breach of a statutory duty. In a "no fault" situation the personal injury insurance will provide a safety net but usually the compensation obtainable is only a small proportion of the amount that would have been awarded by a court in a "fault" situation.

Legal Limitations

Prohibitions on the employment of children of compulsory school age during school hours, etc were removed by the Education (Work Experience) Act 1973 so far as children in their last 12 months of schooling and on official work experience schemes are concerned.

Local by-laws may prohibit employment of children in "undesirable" occupations. These may include work in kitchens, snooker halls, licensed premises, machine arcades, slaughterhouses, dog tracks, race tracks, selling door to door, and window cleaning, except where it is incidental to housework. Such limitations will vary from place to place.

Persons under 18 years of age may not, by virtue of various statutory provisions, be employed in the following situations:

(a) in any process involving asbestos, or in a part of a factory where asbestos dust might enter, or in cleaning protective clothing used in any asbestos process

(b) in blasting processes using sand, shot, grit, etc propelled by compressed air or steam, or to clean such equipment or to be in the vicinity when it is in use (not applicable to construction sites)

(c) in india rubber works, in any fume process in which carbon bisulphide, chloride of sulphur, benzene (or benzol), carbon tetrachloride, trichloroethylene or any carbon chlorine compound is given off

(d) at a furnace where lead or zinc ores are processed, melting scrap lead or zinc, the manufacture of solder or alloys with 10 per cent plus lead, in the manufacture or repair of electric accumulators, where the manipulation of raw oxide of lead is carried on, in the manufacture of lead paints and cleaning areas where lead processes are carried on

(e) in a chemical works in a chrome, nitro or amido process

(f) at any bath or vessel used for electrolytic chromium process

(g) working with radioactive substances including sealed sources and x-ray equipment, or the maintenance of live lasers, microwave or r f emitting equipment

(h) "a young person shall not be employed to lift, carry or move a load so heavy as to be likely to cause injury"

(i) cleaning machines while they are in motion

(j) at heights five metres above ground level or depths below four metres

(k) young women under 18 may not be employed in any lead process or in any part of a factory where the storage of salt or the evaporation of brine in open pans is carried on, or where glass is annealed.

In workplaces subject to the Factories Acts 1961 no young person may operate a prescribed dangerous machine unless fully trained and supervised. These machines are:

(a) brick and tile presses
(b) teasing machines in upholstery or bedding works
(c) carding machines and gill boxes in wool textile trades
(d) corner staying machines
(e) dough brakes
(f) dough mixers
(g) worm pressure extruding machines
(h) hydroextractors, calenders, washing machines and garment presses in laundries
(i) meat mincing machines
(j) pie and tart making machines
(k) power presses, including hydraulic and pneumatic presses
(l) loose knife punching machines
(m) semi-automatic wood turning lathes
(n) guillotine machines
(o) platen printing presses
(p) abrasive wheels and woodworking machines as listed in the Woodworking Machines Regulations 1974.

(Factories Act 1961, s.21).

In premises covered by the Offices, Shops and Railway Premises Act 1963 no person may be put to work on the following specified dangerous machines unless fully instructed in the dangers and precautions to be observed, and operators must be sufficiently trained or, at the very least, work under competent and experienced supervision:

(a) worm type mincers
(b) rotary knife bowl type chopping machines
(c) dough brakes
(d) dough mixers
(e) food mixing machines when used with attachments for mincing, slicing, chipping, or any other cutting operation, or for crumbling
(f) pie and tart making machines
(g) vegetable slicing machines
(h) wrapping and packing machines
(i) garment presses
(j) machines of any type with a circular saw blade

(k) bandsaws
(l) planing machines
(m) vertical spindle moulders
(n) routers

all the above if operated with mechanical power, and the following whether powered or not:

(o) circular knife slicing machines for cutting bacon, etc
(p) potato chipping machines
(q) platen printing machines
(r) guillotine machines.

(Offices, Shops and Railway Premises Act 1963, s.19).

The Pottery (Health and Welfare) Special Regulations 1950 considerably restrict the possible activities of young persons in potteries. Advice should be sought from the local area office of the HSE before pupils are placed in pottery works.

Further reading

Mind How You Go, IND(G) 2L, REV 1990, HSE
The Health and Safety (Training for Employment) Regulations 1990, HMSO
Education at Work—A Guide for Employers, DES 1991
Education at Work—A Guide for Schools, DES 1991

Chapter 20
Information

Providing staff with the information necessary to enable them to carry out their work safely is a requirement of s.2(2) Health and Safety at Work, etc Act 1974 (HASAWA). Each school should set up and maintain a small library of books, booklets, leaflets, etc covering the health and safety aspects of the school's activities.

Such a library should include:

This book
Head's Legal Guide, Croner
Barrel, G R and Partington, J A *Teachers and the Law*, Methuen 1985

DES Safety booklets:
Safety at School: General Advice
Safety in Practical Studies
Safety in Science Laboratories
Safety in Physical Education
Safety in Outdoor Pursuits
(Published by HMSO.)

Association for Science Education booklets:
Safety in the School Laboratory
Topics in Safety
Be Safe (Primary School Science)
(Association for Science Education, College Lane, Hatfield, Hertfordshire AL10 9AA.)

Details of further reading material relevant to specific topics are given throughout this book.

Some LEAs issue bulletins giving information and advice on health and safety issues and where this is the case they should be filed and made available to staff.

Manufacturers and suppliers of articles and substances for use at work are required (s.6 HASAWA) to provide information about such goods to their users. This information should also be collected and included in the library.

The Health and Safety Executive (HSE) Information Services publishes a catalogue of HSC and HSE publications relevant to schools. Free HSE leaflets are available from the HSE Information Centre, Broad Lane, Sheffield SE 7HQ, or via the HSE Freeleaflet Line service, telephone 0742 892346. Priced HSC/HSE publications may be obtained from HMSO.

The Health and Safety Commission publishes a bimonthly newsletter which is distributed by post. For a modest annual cost subscribers receive news about United Kingdom and European health and safety matters, information about new and proposed legislation, reports on accidents and details of new publications. Subscription enquiries should be made to the Publications Department, Room 414, St Hugh's House, Stanley Precinct, Bootle, Merseyside L20 3QY, telephone 051–951 4450.

Further reading

Schools, a list of HSC/E and other relevant publications and films, HSE 1992

'Health and Safety Books from HSE', HMSO Books 1992

Appendix
Reasonable Practicability

Many of the duties imposed on employers by health and safety legislation are qualified by the term "so far as is reasonably practicable". In Chapter 1 a definition is given but it is apparent that most headteachers, safety representatives and others involved in health and safety experience some difficulty in relating this term to practical situations.

The system described below was designed not only to determine whether a proposal for rectification was "reasonably practicable", but also to establish its relative priority. It was used by ILEA safety advisors from 1980 to 1990 to assess thousands of hazards but the subjective element (selecting factor values from tables) requires experience if consistent results are to be obtained. While it is not suggested that staff in schools should use this system rather than seeking the advice of safety officers, consultants or factory inspectors it is worthy of study because of the insight that it gives into the meaning of "reasonable practicability".

The System

The four main factors to be considered when assessing whether a proposal for the rectification of a hazard is reasonably practicable are:

(a) the likely consequences of an accident due to the hazard
(b) the probability of such an accident occurring
(c) the cost of the proposed remedial measures
(d) the degree of correction achievable for that cost.

These factors can be inserted into the equation:

$$\frac{\text{Consequence} \times \text{Probability}}{\text{Cost} \times \text{Degree of Correction}} = \text{Reasonable practicability}$$

When tables are used to give an appropriate numerical value to each factor a number proportional to reasonable practicability is produced.

If the number was 1000 or more immediate action was indicated, with complete isolation of the area of the hazard pending rectification. Between 40 and 1000 the proposed works were reasonably practicable and were expected to be completed within 28 days, during which period any necessary measures to protect site users were applied. Where several proposals were competing for funds the higher the number, the greater was the work's priority. Remedial works scoring less than 40 were not considered to be "reasonably practicable".

It can be seen that while a very expensive option giving 100% correction of a minor hazard may not be reasonably practicable, a cheaper solution giving 80% correction may be legally required.

If "reasonable practicability" in the equation is given the minimum value of 40, simple transposition allows calculation of the expenditure ceiling for rectification of a hazard on strictly legal grounds.

Tables

1. *Degree of Correction*

Degree of correction	Factor value
Hazard totally eliminated	1
75% reduction	1.3
50% reduction	2
25% reduction	4
10% reduction	10

2. *Financial Cost*
Cost of proposed works divided by 1000.

3. *Probability*
Consider frequency of exposure to the hazard, the number of people at risk, any special circumstances such as extra vulnerability of persons at risk, and the degree of intrinsic hazard.

Accident likely with 50% chance of injury once in	Factor value
100 years	7
50 years	13
20 years	29
10 years	50
5 years	75
1 year	100

4. *Consequences*
Assess the most likely outcome of an accident, etc.

	Factor value
Multiple fatalities or major disabling injuries	500
Fatality or major disabling injury	250
Paraplegia or loss of two limbs	200
Severe multiple injuries or extensive burns	120
Total loss of sight	100
Loss or total disablement of hand	70
Permanent minor disablement or disabling illness or loss of an eye	50
Chronic infectious disease (eg Hepatitis B)	30
Loss of thumb	15
Loss of finger	5
Broken leg	3
Broken arm or acute infectious disease (eg dysentery, food poisoning)	2
Severe cuts and bruises	1

(This table was based on the view of the courts of the relative significance of various injuries as demonstrated by the size of compensation awards.)

Main Acts and Statutory Instruments

Acts

1. Education Act 1944
2. Occupier's Liability Act 1957
3. Factories Act 1961
4. Offices, Shops and Railway Premises Act 1963
5. Employer's Liability (Compulsory Insurance) Act 1969
6. Employer's Liability (Defective Equipment) Act 1969
7. Chronically Sick and Disabled Persons Act 1970
8. Fire Precautions Act 1971
9. Employment Medical Advisory Service Act 1972
10. Education (Work Experience) Act 1973
11. Health and Safety at Work, etc Act 1974
12. Employment Protection Act 1975
13. Sex Discrimination Act 1975
14. Congenital Disabilities (Civil Liability) Act 1976
15. Unfair Contract Terms Act 1977
16. Local Government (Miscellaneous Provisions) Act 1982
17. Occupier's Liability Act 1984
18. Social Security Act 1985
19. Public Order Act 1986
20. Consumer Protection Act 1987
21. Education Act 1988
22. Food Safety Act 1990

Statutory Instruments

1. Pottery (Health & Welfare) Special Regulations 1950 (SI 1950 No. 65)
2. Sanitary Accommodation Regulations 1964 (SI 1964 No. 966)
3. Abrasive Wheels Regulations 1970 (SI 1970 No. 535)
4. Woodworking Machines Regulations 1974 (SI 1974 No. 903)
5. Safety Representatives and Safety Committee Regulations 1977 (SI 1977 No. 500)
6. Safety Signs Regulations 1980 (SI 1980 No. 1471)
7. Education (School Premises) Regulations 1981 (SI 1981 No. 909)
8. Health and Safety (First Aid) Regulations 1981 (SI 1981 No. 917)
9. Asbestos (Licensing) Regulations 1983 (SI 1983 No. 1649)
10. Packaging & Labelling of Dangerous Substances Regulations 1984 (SI 1984 No. 1244)
11. Reporting of Injuries, Diseases and Dangerous Occurrences Regulations 1985 (SI 1985 No. 2023)
12. Control of Substances Hazardous to Health Regulations 1988 (SI 1988 No. 1657)
13. Health & Safety (Information for Employees) Regulations 1989 (SI 1989 No. 682)
14. Electricity at Work Regulations 1989 (SI 1989 No. 635)
15. Health & Safety (Training for Employment) Regulations 1990 (SI 1990 No. 1380)
16. Education (School Premises) Amendment Regulations 1990 (SI 1990 No. 2351)
17. Food Hygiene (General) Regulations 1970
18. Traffic Signs Regulations and General Directions 1981
19. Workplace (Health, Safety and Welfare) Regulations 1992
20. Management of Health and Safety at Work Regulations 1992
21. Provision and Use of Work Equipment Regulations 1992
22. Personal Protective Equipment at Work Regulations 1992
23. Health and Safety (Display Screen Equipment) Regulations 1992
24. Manual Handling Operations Regulations 1992
25. Food Premises (Registration) Regulations 1990 and 1991
26. Food Hygiene (Amendment) Regulations 1990

Index